Contents

Topics

Acknowledgements

Contained within the Standard Process and Mediherb formulations are the jewels of nature that when given to the body, enables it to accomplish what is required at a cellular level. Given the proper nutrients, the body is truly its own best pharmacy. It is capable of producing its own remedies such as antibiotics, antidepressants, diuretics, and painkillers. The beauty of the human mechanism is that the dosage is always right and always on time if the cells are properly fed.

Dr. Royal Lee, who founded what today is known as Standard Process Inc, had a vision of what was wrong with the feeding of America. As can be seen from his lectures and writings, Dr. Lee knew of the problems that were occurring during the early part of the twentieth century due to overly processed, nutritionally deficient food. He foresaw what was about to occur in society as a result of this malnutrition. We have seen in this, the twenty-first century, that what he predicted has happened. It was his burning desire to help the undernourished and malnourished that drove him to study and formulate many of the remedies that we have today. When one reads and hears his words, it takes only a few moments to realize that he truly was a visionary. He never thought about limitations, only of what needed to be done for the benefit of mankind. He knew that people were being poisoned by overly processed, adulterated, and synthetically made foodstuffs. He knew that the use of synthetic molecules by themselves could not and would not restore normal physiology. He saw the nutritional castration that was occurring and the problems with the nutritional supplement industry. He had a message to tell, and it is to perpetuate his vision, that this manual was created.

Associate Professor Kerry Bone, the founder of MediHerb, is another visionary. He saw the inconsistencies that were common in the herbal industry. His desire to produce accurate literature and quality herbal products is testament to his desire to help remedy human suffering. His ability to take nature's bounty and transform it into potent herbal medicine is truly a gift to humanity.

I owe a depth of gratitude to Dr. Royal Lee and Kerry Bone. For without them many sick and malnourished people would be without help. The potent whole food nutrition and herbal medicines they have pioneered have provided me with the tools I need in order to make available what so many people need so desperately, potent whole food nutrition and herbal medicines.

I would like to thank Joseph Olejak, D.C. for his resilience, patience, and contribution to this project. You have my utmost respect and gratitude.

To the following individuals I am also deeply indebted. Your input regarding clinical expertise, product knowledge, patience with me, and help in putting together the text is sincerely appreciated. Without your knowledge and support none of this would of have been possible.

- Angela Hywood ND.
- Amanda Williams ND.
- Associate Professor Kerry Bone B.Sc. (Hons), Dip Phyto, FNIMH, FHHAA, MCPP
- Bruce Poritzky
- Linda Ryan ND., AHG
- Mark Anderson
- Tim Bahan

Your dedication to this project will help many people in need. For this you should be proud.

I also would like to thank Jackie Fett for her editing of the text. My constant tweaking of the material and her patience with me in doing this is and always will be appreciated.

To all involved, once again, thank you,

Bruce Bond D.C.

Introduction

Synergistic Therapeutics:
Combining Whole Food Nutrition and Herbal Medicines for Common Ailments

Introduction

As practitioners, we find ourselves having to decide how to best address the problems that plague our patients. They present us with varied symptoms that usually have terminology ascribed to them that in turn is labeled as a diagnosis of a condition.

We understand that behind the diagnosis is a history of causes and effects which collectively we call etiology. The mystery practitioners need to solve is: What nutritional and herbal supplementation is needed to best support normal physiological and biochemical processes to foster the natural healing mechanism?

Synergistic Therapeutics provides some of those answers. This manual brings together Standard Process® whole food supplements and MediHerb® herbal products in a format that will enable you to provide the nutritional support needed by those individuals, with the conditions listed herein. Both Standard Process and MediHerb are available only through health care professionals. In terms of quality and therapeutic benefits, these products provide consistent results in clinical practice. Standard Process grows the majority of raw materials on company-owned, certified organic farmland, and MediHerb uses a unique method of extraction, termed Cold Percolation. Visit www.standardprocess.com to learn more about Standard Process and MediHerb.

This reference manual explains how to support the natural healing process using the 'functional components' found in whole foods and herbs. It emphasizes the importance of long-term wellness instead of short-term symptomatic changes.

This text is useful to the practitioner because it combines a concise description of each ailment with symptoms, etiology, and suggestions for nutritional support in a well-organized and easy-to-implement format.

In addition, the organization of this book builds confidence in nutritional and herbal prescribing by giving physiological information about each product suggested. Understanding those connections are important when facing each person's unique health history. It is for this reason that some protocols may need to be adjusted, based on clinical judgment, for the best "fit" for individual patients.

The prescribing approach is consistent throughout, and each topic builds on the next. Whole foods and herbs were purposefully combined in this text because of the interaction between these two kinds of plants. This adds yet another layer of synergy on top of the beneficial effects gained by using whole plants instead of isolated components.

Knowledge from clinical practice and reference to research makes this book both authoritative and easy to use. We hope you will continually use this information as a resource in your clinical practice.

When reading each section, please remember:

1. The primary protocol should be used in its entirety.

2. The secondary protocol is adjunctive therapy. This means that you should pick the products that you feel may benefit your patient <u>in addition</u> to the primary protocol. Any one or a combination of them may be considered.

It is our pleasure to present this manual. Our purpose is to make a positive difference in people's lives with the information found within its pages.

In health,

Bruce Bond, DC   Joseph Olejak, DC

Catalyn® (Multivitamin)

Catalyn was the first product developed by Dr. Royal Lee in 1929. The production of this multivitamin also marked the beginning of the company which is now known as Standard Process Inc. Dr. Lee spent many years researching a whole food based supplement, using vitamins and minerals in their natural state, as opposed to parts of the whole food complex. Dr. Lee knew there was a need for Catalyn because of the modern diet and over consumption of processed and nutritionally deficient foods.

It is important to remember that in addition to the particular protocol you recommend for your adult patients, they should also be given at least six Catalyn (multivitamin) per day and four Linum B6 (Standard Process) for essential fatty acids (EFAs).

The reason for recommending Catalyn® and EFAs is to ensure that the baseline nutritional status of the patient is adequate for optimal healing to take place. For example, let's assume you were giving adrenal gland support and utilizing only the products under the primary support in the adrenal section. The patient may now have excellent adrenal support and the glands may be functioning better, but what about the nutritional status of the other organs? Perhaps there is some missing nutrient(s) not supplied by the adrenal support, or by the patient's diet. Catalyn is the best general support available. With its known and unknown nutrients only found in whole food complexes, Catalyn is truly the complete multivitamin. By providing your patients with Catalyn and the essential fatty acids (essential because the body cannot manufacture them), you can be sure your patient has the best chance for a positive clinical response.

Think of Catalyn as the catalyst of healing. Like any catalyst, it promotes a normal process that might otherwise move ahead at a much slower pace.

Preface

There is no greater privilege than being entrusted with the health care of another human being. It is also an honor to be in a position to educate new generations of healthcare providers and to further the work of those of the past. I again would like to thank all those involved who have generously contributed their time, energy, and talents to this text. In doing so, they will be helping many more patients than they could ever physically see. Finally, I urge all health care providers to be lifelong students, because as clinicians, this is a responsibility we owe to those who put their trust in our hands.

Bruce Bond D.C.

Reader Information and Disclaimer

The concepts and principles herein relate to the promotion and maintenance of health, not the diagnosis or treatment of disease related to physical and/or emotional complaints.

The information in this book is not intended as suggestions for self-diagnosis or self-treatment of mental, emotional, or physical symptoms or ailments. The information contained within provides an overview of the topics discussed, however one should remember that for a complete review of the topic and information discussed, the appropriate texts should be consulted. The notes are intended for use by experienced professional clinicians with a background of education and experience in physiology. Without experience, the notes can be misunderstood, misapplied, and/or abused. The authors take no responsibility for the misapplication of the information in these notes. Results of any product usage may vary.

This book deals with Synergistic Therapeutics — the use of whole food nutrition and herbal medicines to support normal physiology — and certain elements of lifestyle can have a strong influence on physiology.

Any references in the text to specific conditions do not infer treatment for these conditions. The description of any condition within these notes is for description and educational purposes only. The authors are not implying treatments for diseases. Any use of nutritional supplements or herbs is simply given in the context of supplying nutritional and/or herbal support for those with a said condition or without said condition.

No guarantee or assurance of any specific result is given or implied from any suggestions or recommendations herein.

The reader is reminded that regular examinations for the early detection of disease are important.

The publisher and authors are not responsible for factual errors, inaccuracies, or omissions although every effort has been made to use the most current information available.

The statements contained within this manual have not been evaluated by the Food & Drug Administration. The products referenced to and recommendations put forth are not intended to diagnose, treat, cure, or prevent any disease. Specific product names have been used to simplify for the clinician the implementation of the principles discussed herein. Any mention of any specific product is the opinion of the authors and not that of the company which produced said products.

Additionally, the publisher and authors disclaim any adverse reactions or consequences arising out of the use of any of the suggestions, preparations, or procedures discussed in this book.

All matters pertaining to physical and emotional health should be supervised by a duly qualified health care professional.

Practitioners are advised to consult appropriate texts for any contraindications regarding usage of both Standard Process® and MediHerb® products and for additional in-depth review of the conditions discussed here within.

Adrenal Insufficiency

Defined

Adrenal Insufficiency (also known as adrenal fatigue) involves damaged, overworked, or depleted adrenal glands.

Signs and Symptoms

The adrenal glands are actually two separate endocrine glands each consisting of a medulla and cortex. Each gland produces its own hormones (described below). It is easier to understand the ramifications of adrenal fatigue if one is aware of the physiologic roles played by these two glands. With this in mind, the following review should bring to light the diverse symptomatology that can result from adrenal fatigue.

Adrenal Medulla

Cells in the adrenal medulla synthesize and secrete epinephrine and norepinephrine. The principal actions of these two hormones are to:

- Increase the heart rate and force of contraction
- Cause widespread vasoconstriction resulting in increased resistance to blood flow and hence arterial blood pressure
- Cause bronchial dilation
- Stimulate lipolysis in fat cells
- Increase cellular oxygen consumption
- Stimulate the release of stored glycogen from the liver to raise blood sugar between meals and during periods of increased physiologic demands
- Inhibit digestion
- Dilate the pupils

Adrenal Cortex

The adrenal cortex is the site of steroid hormone production. The cortex secretes three types of steroid hormones: mineralocorticoids, glucocorticoids, and sex hormones. Sex hormones, such as estrogens and androgens, are produced in very small amounts.

Physiologic Effects of Mineralocorticoids

Aldosterone
Aldosterone is a mineralocorticosteroid hormone synthesized and secreted by (the zona glomerulosa of) the adrenal cortex of the adrenal glands.

- Increased resorption of sodium in the distal tubules of the kidneys
- Increased resorption of water which is an osmotic effect related to its effect on sodium
- Increased renal excretion of potassium

Cortisol
This hormone stimulates several processes that collectively increase and maintain normal concentrations of glucose in the blood. These effects include:

- Stimulating gluconeogenesis, particularly in the liver using substrates such as lipids and amino acids
- Mobilizes and increases amino acids in the blood and liver
- Stimulating glycogen formation in the liver
- Mobilizing and increases fatty acids and glycerol in the blood to be used as fuel for energy production

6

Adrenal Insufficiency

- Inhibiting glucose uptake in muscle and adipose tissue thus keeping blood glucose levels elevated enabling the body to meet its cellular energy requirements during periods of stress.
- Countering inflammation and in excess can suppress immune function
- Preventing the loss of sodium in the urine thus helping to maintain blood pressure and volume

DHEA
Dehydroepiandrosterone (DHEA) is a hormone manufactured primarily in the adrenal cortex of the adrenal glands. DHEA is also produced in small amounts by individual neurons in the brain. DHEA is the most abundant steroid hormone in the bloodstream.

- Functions as an androgen with anabolic activity (builder of tissue)
- Precursor to testosterone
- Precursor to estrogen(s)
- Reverses immune suppression caused by excess cortisol levels, thus improving resistance to bacterial, viral, and parasitic infection.
- Works inversely with cortisol
- Increases muscle mass, decreases percent body fat
- Lowers total cholesterol and LDL levels

Etiology

There are many causes of adrenal fatigue, some common examples are:

- Stress: This can be emotional (anxiety, depression, etc.) and or physical (e.g., chronic illness, change of season, excessive exercise)
- Nutritional deficiency
- Excess refined carbohydrate intake
- Excessive use of caffeine
- Alcohol
- Nicotine
- Surgery
- Toxin exposure
- Menopause
- Pregnancy

Supplementation

Primary Support

Note: The following will provide you with two alternatives with which to provide adrenal support. Protocol I is the Standard Process program and Protocol II the Mediherb program. In practice, I always like to feed the body with nutritional products and utilize the herbs as adjuncts when needed. You will need to determine which is best in your particular patient's case. Do not hesitate to use products from both product lines, such as utilizing Withania Complex along with Drenamin® and Cataplex® B.

Protocol I

Drenamin® (Standard Process): Supplies Cataplex® C (the adrenals utilize and store the largest amount of vitamin C as compared to any other gland in the body) and adrenal Protomorphogen™ extract support along with Cataplex® G to provide the B vitamins, which are needed to ensure optimal oxygen delivery to the tissues.

Dosage: Two to three tablets, three times per day with meals.

Cataplex® B (Standard Process): The B complex vitamins contained in this formula complement Drenamin® so as to supply all the B vitamins needed to ensure optimal ATP production at the cellular level. The thiamine in this formula is critical in order to facilitate the conversion of pyruvic acid to acetyl-CoA to support maximum ATP production in the mitochondria.

Dosage: Two tablets, three times per day with meals.

Note: By giving Drenamin® and Cataplex® B, the entire vitamin B complex is supplied to the body.

Protocol II

Withania Complex (MediHerb): Formula for those who are "wired up" and "run down" at the same time. This formula combines the effects of Licorice, Withania, Skullcap and Korean Ginseng.

Dosage: One tablet, three to four times per day.

Licorice High Grade 1:1 (MediHerb) or Rehmannia 1:2 (MediHerb): Adrenal trophorestoratives.

Dosage: Licorice High Grade 1:1 – Four mL per day.
Rehmannia 1:2 – Seven mL per day.

Eleuthero 1:2 (Siberian ginseng): General adaptogenic support and adrenal tonic.

Dosage: One tablet three times per day or two to four mL of liquid extract once or twice per day.

Anemia (Iron Deficiency & Pernicious)

Defined

Anemia is a reduction in the oxygen-carrying capacity of the blood as a result of a deficiency in the quantity of red blood cells or hemoglobin in the blood.

Iron deficiency anemia (Hypochromic-Microcytic Anemia) is the result of insufficient iron availability, resulting in reduced hemoglobin production.

Pernicious anemia (Megaloblastic Macrocytic Anemia) results from a deficiency of intrinsic factor (a small glyco-protein secreted by the gastric mucosa which is responsible for transporting vitamin B12 to the ileum for absorption), which in turn leads to a vitamin B12 deficiency.

Signs and Symptoms

Iron Deficiency Anemia

- Pallor
- Weakness
- Irritability
- Fatigue
- Drowsiness
- Difficulty in concentration and learning impairment
- Cravings for non foods (pica), such as dirt and ice
- Spoon nails
- Leg cramps at night
- Cold extremities
- Reduced immune function
- In severe cases, anemia may cause headaches, tinnitus, digestive upset, dizziness, spots before the eyes, and a rapid heart beat

Pernicious Anemia

- Anorexia
- Intermittent diarrhea and constipation
- Diffuse abdominal pain
- Burning of the tongue
- Considerable weight loss
- Ataxia
- Irritability
- Loss of positional and vibratory sensation in the extremities accompanied with moderate weakness and reflex loss.
- Mild depression
- Yellow blue blindness
- Confusion
- Postural hypotension
- Delirium

Etiology

Iron Deficiency Anemia

- Blood loss through menstruation
- Bleeding hemorrhoids
- Gastrointestinal lesions
- Weak exocrine pancreatic functioning
- Decreased iron absorption
- Pregnancy (increased iron need by mother)
- Chronic antacid use
- Bleeding ulcers
- Nutritional deficiencies of vitamin B12, folic acid, and/or iron
- Inadequate gastric production of hydrochloric acid
- Lack of intrinsic factor
- Iron deficiency anemia in vegetarianism
- Chronic diarrhea (iron deficiency anemia)

Pernicious Anemia

- Veganism: Nutritional deficiency.
- Inadequate absorption: Lack of intrinsic factor (pernicious anemia, endocrinopathy, destruction of the gastric mucosa) and small intestine disorders (e.g. celiac disease, malignancy, vitamin B12 malabsorption, and competition for B12 such as with fish tapeworm and blind loop syndrome).

Anemia (Iron Deficiency & Pernicious)

- Inadequate utilization: Enzyme deficiencies, transport protein abnormality, organ disease (liver, kidney, malnutrition, or malignancy).
- Increased requirement: Infancy, hyperthyroidism, and parasitic infestation.
- Increased excretion: Inadequate binding in serum, liver disease, and kidney disease.

Treatment Considerations

Once a clinical evaluation has determined which form of anemia is present, one can then formulate a strategy regarding nutritional and herbal support. The following sections will help you formulate a protocol that is most appropriate for your patient.

Supplementation

Choose from either Protocol I or Protocol II when providing nutritional or herbal support for both Iron Deficiency Anemia and Pernicious Anemia.

Primary Support: Protocol I

Ferrofood® (Standard Process): Supplies not only ferrous lactate, which is a very assimilable form of iron, but also other synergistic factors to help ensure optimal red blood cell production and removal.

Dosage: One capsule, three times per day with meals.

Folic Acid B12 (Standard Process): Each tablet supplies 100% of the RDA of folic acid and B12 along with other synergistic cofactors such as desiccated stomach to provide the intrinsic factor needed to support absorption of vitamin B12.

Dosage: One to two tablets, three times per day with meals.

Chlorophyll Complex™ (Standard Process): Traditionally used as a blood builder due to the chlorophyll molecule having a similar molecular structure to hemoglobin, the core mineral is magnesium in place of iron. Chlorophyll perles are also an excellent source of the fat-soluble vitamin factors.

Dosage: Two perles, three times per day with meals.

Zypan® (Standard Process): In patients with compromised gastric digestion, the addition of this formula will facilitate the assimilation of iron. Zypan® supplies betaine hydrochloride, pepsin, ammonium chloride along with pancreatic enzymes to support optimal protein, fat, and carbohydrate digestion. Consider this the chief Standard Process proteolytic product with some broad based small intestinal digestive support and acidifying factors needed to ensure optimal gastric pH.

Dosage: One to two tablets, three times a day with meals.

Primary Support: Protocol II

Fe-Max Iron Tonic Phytosynergist™ (MediHerb): Non-alcohol based herbal formula which supports normal red blood cell production, encourages healthy digestion, and is a source of iron and B vitamins, including vitamin B12 and folic acid. Vegetarian alternative to Ferrofood®

Dosage: Five mL, three times per day.

DiGest Phytosynergist™ (MediHerb): A bitter herbal formula which enhances hydrochloric acid secretion, acts as a choleretic, and stimulates the release of pancreatic amylase, lipase, and protease.

Dosage: Five mL, fifteen to twenty minutes prior to meals.

Anemia (Iron Deficiency & Pernicious)

Secondary Support

Considering the role that bone tissue has in red blood cell production the following products can be valuable adjuncts in certain cases. Choose the product(s) that best meet the needs of the case in question.

Ostrophin PMG® (Standard Process): Source of bone Protomorphogen™ extract and whole veal bone components.

Dosage: One to two tablets, three times per day with meals.

Bio-Dent® (Standard Process): Supplies the nutrients that are needed to support optimal bone health. Since it does not have any Protomorphogen™ extracts in it, using it along with Ostrophin PMG® provides a synergistic formula to support optimal bone rebuilding.

Dosage: Five tablets, three times per day with meals.

Anxiety

Defined

Generalized anxiety disorder is the excessive, usually daily, worry and nervousness about a variety of events or activities.

Signs and Symptoms

- Constantly worried or distressed (the frequency, duration, and anxiety of the worries is disproportionately greater than the situation warrants)
- Restlessness
- Fatigue easily
- Irritability
- Muscular tension
- Disturbed sleep
- Palpitations or accelerated heart rate
- Difficulty concentrating
- Difficulty sleeping
- Excessive behavior (abuse of alcohol or food, etc.)
- Bowel dysfunction (e.g. constipation, diarrhea)

Etiology

- Caffeine; either from excessive intake or withdrawal
- Nicotine withdrawal
- Excessive consumption of Ephedrine
- Excessive accumulation of endogenous lactic acid
- Nutritional deficiencies
- Pharmaceutical drug use
- Anxiety can be the result of PMS
- Food additives
- Environmental toxins
- Systemic Candida albicans
- Hypoglycemia
- Hypothyroidism
- Adrenal insufficiency
- Impaired circulation to the brain
- Excessive copper and/or mercury body burden
- Biochemical abnormalities of brain chemistry
- Emotional stress
- Food intolerance/allergies
- Lack of sleep

Treatment Considerations

- Use of sedative and anxiolytic remedies
- Use of parasympathetic support remedies to balance an overactive sympathetic response
- Use of nutritional and Protomorphogen™ extract support should be considered with adrenal exhaustion as a result of prolonged sympathetic stimulation

Supplementation

Primary Support

Min-Chex® (Standard Process): Contains calcium, magnesium, kelp, Niacinamide B6, orchic Cytosol™ extract along with those nutrients that function synergistically to support the parasympathetic nervous system and enhance oxygen delivery to the brain.

Dosage: Two capsules, three times per day with meals.

Anxiety

Note: An excellent alternative to Min-Chex® is **Min-Tran®** (Standard Process). Min-Tran® is chiefly composed of calcium lactate, magnesium, kelp and alfalfa. It is higher in calcium and magnesium than Min-Chex®, but does not contain the orchic Cytosol™ extract or Niacinamide B6. Min-Tran® could be considered a mineral tranquilizer.

Dosage: Three to four tablets three times per day with meals.

Drenamin® (Standard Process): A special formula of Cataplex® C, Cataplex® G, adrenal Protomorphogen™ extract, and other vital nutrients which help maintain healthy functioning adrenal glands.

Dosage: Two to three tablets, three times per day with meals.

Valerian Complex (MediHerb): The combination of Valerian root, Passion flower, and Valerian root and rhizome makes this product effective for those dealing with stress and anxiety.

Dosage: Three to four tablets per day.

Asthma

Defined

Asthma is defined as a condition characterized by recurrent attacks of paroxysmal, reversible airway obstruction, airway inflammation, and increased airway responsiveness to a variety of stimuli.

Asthma can be classified as either extrinsic or intrinsic and each classification has a different set of triggers. Extrinsic asthma is caused by some factor in the environment, usually allergic asthma. Intrinsic asthma is attributed to some pathophysiologic disturbance and not an environmental factor(s).

Signs and Symptoms

- Wheezing
- Coughing
- Difficulty breathing

Etiology

Asthma can result from sensitivity to intrinsic or extrinsic allergens. Patients with intrinsic, or nonatopic asthma react to internal, nonallergenic factors; external substances cannot be implicated in patients with intrinsic asthma. The majority of episodes occur after a severe respiratory infection.

Intrinsic allergens include:

- Emotional stress, anxiety
- Irritants
- Endocrine changes
- Fatigue
- Humidity and temperature variations
- Genetic factors
- Coughing or laughing

Extrinsic or atopic asthma typically begins in childhood; patients are sensitive to specific external allergens.

Extrinsic allergens include:

- Animal dander
- Pollen
- Mold or house dust
- Feather pillows
- Food additives, including some dyes and sulfites
- Noxious fumes

Many asthmatics have both intrinsic and extrinsic asthma.

Treatment Considerations

Some of the goals practitioners will want to achieve with natural remedies are:

- Control the allergic response
- Address sinusitis
- Clear airways
- Improve digestion
- Eliminate infection
- Balance immunity
- Improve mucus membrane function and tone
- Moderate the effects of stress
- Reduce catarrh (mucus production)
- Reduce local inflammation

Supplementation

Primary Support

ResCo® (MediHerb): A combination herbal product containing licorice, mullein, euphorbia, grindelia, ginger, and fennel. ResCo helps to soothe inflamed mucous membranes, reduce coughing, remove mucus, dilate airways, and stimulate circulation.

Asthma

Dosage: Acute conditions - Two tablets, three times per day.
Chronic conditions - One tablet, three times per day.

Pneumotrophin PMG® (Standard Process): Support for the lungs utilizing lung Protomorphogen™ extract.

Dosage: One tablet, three times per day with meals.

Cataplex® A-C (Standard Process): The vitamin A and C complex factors found in Cataplex A-C are needed for the maintenance and health of the mucous membranes, optimal tissue restoration, and immune support. Without these factors or nutrients these tissues become susceptible to pollution, infections, irritation, catarrhal states, and allergies. The vitamin C complex is essential to the adrenal glands normal function since they utilize and store a tremendous amount of vitamin C complex.

Dosage: Three tablets, three times per day with meals.

Drenatrophin PMG® (Standard Process): Provides adrenal Protomorphogen™ extract. The adrenal glands (better known as the stress glands) are susceptible to fatigue under a chronic allergic response.

Dosage: Two tablets, two times per day with meals.

Echinacea Premium (MediHerb): Immune enhancement using a combination of *Echinacea angustifolia* and *Echinacea purpurea* root.

Dosage: One tablet, three times per day.

Secondary Support: As Indicated

As the etiology above suggests, asthma is a condition that has a variety of clinical presentations. Use the guide below to determine which secondary support is indicated.

Asthma with bacterial/viral sinusitis: Refer to the section titled *Sinusitis*.

Asthma with poor digestion: Refer to the section titled *Inadequate Digestion*.

Asthma associated with anxiety and/or depression: Refer to the sections titled *Anxiety and Depression*.

Asthma with excess mucus production: Fen-Gre® (Standard Process) - Three to five capsules two to three times per day with a large glass of water.

Asthma with Chronic Dry Cough: Marshmallow Root 1:5 Glycetract (MediHerb) - Five mL three to four times daily or as needed.

Asthma with Hypothalamus-Pituitary-Adrenal (HPA) axis overlay: Symplex® M for males and Symplex® F for females.

Symplex® M (Standard Process): Male endocrine support including the Protomorphogens™ of the pituitary, thyroid, adrenal glands, and testicles.

Dosage: One to two tablets, three times daily with meals.

Symplex® F (Standard Process): Female endocrine support including the Protomorphogens™ of the pituitary, thyroid, adrenal glands, and ovaries.

Dosage: One to two tablets, three times daily with meals.

Hypothalamus PMG™ (Standard Process): Protomorphogen™ extract support for the hypothalamus.

Dosage: One to two tablets, three times daily with meals.

Benign Prostatic Hyperplasia (BPH)

Defined

Benign prostatic hyperplasia (BPH) is a benign (non-cancerous) enlargement of the periurethral prostate gland, resulting in differing degrees of bladder outlet obstruction. Based on histological diagnosed BPH from autopsy studies, the incidence increases from 8% in men aged 31 to 40 years old to 40-50% in men aged 51 to 60 years old. The incidence is greater than 80% in men older then 80 years old. Based on these results, it is clear that BPH becomes increasingly more prevalent as men age, especially after the age of 50.

Signs and Symptoms

- Progressive urinary urgency, frequency, and nocturia as a result of incomplete emptying and refilling of the bladder
- Reduced size and force of the urinary stream can result in hesitancy and intermittency
- Feeling of incomplete emptying, terminal dribbling, incontinence, or complete urinary retention may ensue

Etiology

- Age related hormonal changes. In the aging male, testosterone levels have been shown to decrease while the levels of estrogen increase.
- Increased levels of 5-alpha dihydrotestosterone (DHT), the most active metabolite of testosterone, appears to be a major etiological factor in the development of BPH.
- High estrogen levels in the male have been implicated in increasing the conversion of testosterone to 5-alpha dihydrotestosterone and/or inhibiting the elimination of DHT from the prostate. If this is the case, then the exposure to xenoestrogens could be a causative factor in the development of BPH.
- High blood cholesterol levels correlated with high prostate cholesterol levels have been cited as a possible cause of BPH.
- Nutritional deficiency (e.g. zinc, lycopene, vitamins A, D, E).
- Inadequate hepatic detoxification of hormones due to poor liver function.

Treatment Considerations

Nutritional and herbal protocols should:

- Inhibit 5-alpha-reductase
- Reduce edema
- Control inflammation
- Provide nutritional and Protomorphogen™ extract support for the prostate tissue

Clinicians are advised to consider sub-clinical kidney involvement when BPH is formally diagnosed. Left untreated, BPH can lead to the eventual obstruction of urine flow from the bladder resulting in urine retention and potential kidney damage at the cellular level.

Benign Prostatic Hyperplasia (BPH)

Supplementation

Primary Protocol

Cataplex® F Tablets (Standard Process): The formula has provided an observed effect of benefiting those with BPH do its ability to help diffuse calcium ions into tissues.

Dosage: Four tablets, three times per day with meals.

Zinc Liver Chelate™ (Standard Process): Zinc has been shown to be of benefit for an enlarged prostate by inhibiting the 5-Alpha Reductase enzyme that is responsible for the conversion of testosterone to dihydrotestosterone.

Dosage: Two tablets, twice per day with meals for one month; upon completion, switch to:

Chezyn® (Standard Process): A balanced supplement of iron, copper, and zinc.

Dosage: Two to three tablets, three times per day with meals.

Note: Consider utilization of Standard Process' Zinc Test™. This is a non-invasive way to determine a patient's zinc status.

Serenoa Complex (MediHerb): This complex is in a pumpkin seed oil base. The active constituents of saw palmetto are lipophilic, hence the oil base. Pumpkin seed oil is a rich source of zinc and essential fatty acids. Traditional known actions include anti-inflammatory, mild diuretic, and antispasmodic.

Dosage: Serenoa Complex - Two to three tablets per day.

Prostate PMG® (Standard Process): Prostate support utilizing Protomorphogen™ extract.

Dosage: One to two tablets, three times per day with meals.

Nettle Root 1:2 (MediHerb): Has an effect on dihydrotestosterone and epidermal growth factor resulting in reducing inflammation and enhancing urinary flow.

Dosage: Seven mL per day.

Secondary Protocol: As Indicated

Horsechestnut Complex (MediHerb): Anti-inflammatory and anti-edema formula.

Dosage: One tablet, three times per day with meals.

Prost-X™ (Standard Process): Support for the prostate utilizing prostate Cytosol™ extract.

Dosage: One capsule, three times per day with meals.

Cranberry Complex (MediHerb): Demulcent and antiseptic support for any accompanying urinary tract infection.

Dosage: Two to three tablets, two times per day.

Cramplex (MediHerb): The herbs in Cramplex provide antispasmodic activity to ease occasional spasms of smooth muscle which may be of benefit with BPH.

Dosage: One to two tablets, two times per day.

Note: Both the primary and secondary protocols can be used long term.

Bronchitis (Acute)

Defined

Acute inflammation of the tracheobronchial tree. Commonly mild, however, acute bronchitis can be serious in patients with chronic lung or heart disease and in debilitated patients. Airflow obstruction is a common sequalae, and pneumonia can be a serious complication. Symptoms that last up to 90 days are usually classified as acute bronchitis while symptoms lasting longer are usually classified as chronic bronchitis.

Signs and Symptoms

- The initial onset of bronchitis is an unproductive and often painful cough, which progresses to the increased production of mucus culminating in an infection. An infection starting in the trachea can progress into the bronchi.
- Fever of 100° to 102° F (37.8° to 38.9° C).
- The sputum in acute bronchitis is typically green or yellow, whereas the sputum in chronic bronchitis is grey or white.

Etiology and Predisposing Factors

Acute bronchitis can be the result of an infection or exposure to irritants.

Acute Infectious Bronchitis

- Most often caused by viruses.
- Bacterial infection commonly develops after a common cold or viral infection of the throat, tracheobronchial tree, or nasopharynx.
- Malnutrition increases the risk of upper respiratory tract infections and the resulting acute bronchitis.
- Chronic sinus infections and allergies increase the likelihood of repeated episodes of acute bronchitis.
- Those with chronic lung diseases and smokers have an increased incidence of repeated attacks of acute bronchitis due to the inability of mucus to be expelled from the airways.

Acute Irritative Bronchitis

- Inhaled irritants such as strong acids and certain volatile organic solvents such as ammonia, chlorine, sulfur dioxide, and tobacco smoke.

Treatment Considerations

- Enhance immune function with appropriate nutritional support
- Provide nutritional support specific to the respiratory system
- Employ diaphoretic remedies where fever is involved
- Anticatarrhal remedies
- Antitussive support

Supplementation

Primary Support

Broncafect® or Broncafect Phytosynergist™ (both MediHerb): Provides immune enhancing, mucolytic, expectorant, bronchodilatory, and diaphoretic activity.

Bronchitis (Acute)

Dosage: Broncafect® – Two tablets, three times per day until the bottle is finished.
> Or
> Broncafect Phytosynergist™ – Five mL, three to four times per day until the bottle is finished.

Congaplex® (Standard Process): Combines the vitamin C and A complex factors, thymus Cytosol™ extract, calcium lactate, and cellular protein precursor material in the form of RNA. This formula provides the nutrients and tissue extracts that contribute to an efficient response by the immune system.

Dosage: Four capsules, three times per day. Consider using three to four capsules per hour for four to six hours and then reduce the dosage to four capsules three times per day as the symptoms subside. Have the patient continue at this dosage until the bottle is finished.

Andrographis Complex (MediHerb): Provides additional immune stimulating, immune modulating, and antipyretic activity via the combination of the following herbs: *Echinacea angustifolia,* Holy Basil, and Andrographis.

Dosage: Two tablets, three to four times per day.

Pneumotrophin PMG® (Standard Process): Lung Protomorphogen™ extract helps maintain the lungs in a good state of repair to support healthy respiratory function.

Dosage: Two tablets, three times per day with meals.

Cal-Amo® (Standard Process): The acidifying compounds in this formula such as ammonium chloride and betaine hydrochloride support proper acid/alkaline balance in the respiratory tissues which indirectly will optimize the immune response.

Dosage: One tablet, three times per day with meals.

Have the patient finish all of the above remedies. If clinically indicated, all of the following or any combination thereof can be used for long term prophylaxis.

- **Pneumotrophin PMG® (Standard Process):** Two tablets, three times per day with meals.
- **Immuplex® (Standard Process):** Provides the vitamin A, C, and E complexes, folic acid, cyanocobalamin, trace minerals, and liver, thymus, spleen, and bone Protomorphogen™ extracts along with other synergistic factors for optimal immune system support. This is not a product to be used for an acute case but rather for those with depleted immune systems that require the nutritional factors to optimize the immune response. Two to three capsules, three times per day with meals.

- **Cataplex® C (Standard Process):** Provides the vitamin C and A complexes, trace minerals, and associated nutrients to support optimal immune responsiveness. Two to three tablets, three times per day with meals.

Secondary Support: As Indicated

DiaCo Phytosynergist™ (MediHerb): Diaphoretic formula that can be used as a:

- Anti-infective
- Immune enhancer
- Diaphoretic
- Demulcent
- Anticatarrhal
- Expectorant

Dosage: Five mL, three to five times per day with a small glass of warm water until fever subsides, then discontinue. Can be sipped as a tea.

Note: Since this is a diaphoretic formula it is to be used only if fever is present.

Bronchitis (Acute)

Cataplex® A-C (Standard Process): Provides the vitamin A and C complex factors to support the immune system as well as the maintenance of healthy epithelial and connective tissues.

Dosage: Two tablets, three times per day with meals.

Calcium Lactate (Standard Process): Source of ionizable and diffusible calcium to support optimal phagocyte activity.

Dosage: Two tablets, three times per day. Best taken one hour before or two hours after meals.

Golden Seal 500mg (MediHerb): Provides antimicrobial, antibacterial, vulnerary, and mucous membrane trophorestorative actions. Golden Seal is particularly useful for catarrhal states of the mucous membranes.

Dosage: One tablet, three times per day.

Echinacea Premium (MediHerb): Immune modulating.

Dosage: One tablet, three times per day.

Garlic *(Organically Grown)* **(Standard Process):** Provides antimicrobial and mucolytic activity.

Dosage: One capsule, three times per day with meals.

Marshmallow Root 1:5 Glycetract: Provides demulcent activity which is useful for irritations of the oral and pharyngeal mucosa, dry cough, and chronic irritable cough.

Dosage: Three mL, once or twice per day.

Bronchitis (Chronic)

Defined

Form of bronchitis characterized by a chronic productive cough that is present for at least three months of two consecutive years when other causes such as infections, lung carcinoma, or chronic heart failure have been ruled out.

Signs and Symptoms

- Abundance of gray, white, or yellow sputum
- Tachypnea, dyspnea
- Pedal edema
- Cyanosis
- Neck vein distention
- Weight gain due to edema
- Weight loss due to increased metabolic rate or edema
- Pulmonary hypertension
- Prolonged expiratory time and/or wheezing

Etiology

- Exposure to irritants
- Cigarette smoke
- Exposure to noxious gases
- Genetic predisposition
- Respiratory tract infection
- Exposure to inorganic or organic dusts

Treatment Considerations

- Employ the use of mucolytic, expectorant, bronchodilating, and anticatarrhal agents as needed
- Enhance immune function
- Utilize respiratory antiseptics
- Offer heart support, if indicated

Supplementation

Primary Support

ResCo® or ResCo Phytosynergist™ (MediHerb): Provides the following actions: expectorant, demulcent, antispasmodic, and anti-inflammatory.

Dosage: **ResCo®** – Four to six tablets per day.
　　　　Or
　　　　ResCo Phytosynergist™ – Five mL, three times per day.

} Duration of use is six weeks on and two week off, etc.

Echinacea Premium (MediHerb): To enhance the immune response.

Dosage: Two to three tablets per day.

Bronchitis (Chronic)

Pneumotrophin PMG® (Standard Process): Lung support utilizing Protomorphogen™ extracts.

Dosage: One tablet, three times per day with meals.

Garlic *(Organically Grown)* (Standard Process): Provides antimicrobial and mucolytic activity.

Dosage: One capsule, three times per day with meals.

Note: Primary support can be used long term as described.

Secondary Support: As Indicated

Fen-Gre® (Standard Process): Source of fenugreek seed powder which has a thinning effect on mucus. Fen-Gre helps the body to expel mucus and phlegm from the bronchial tubes.

Dosage: Three capsules, three times per day with a full glass of water.

Golden Seal 500mg (MediHerb): Provides antimicrobial, antibacterial, vulnerary, and mucous membrane trophorestorative actions.

Dosage: One tablet, three times per day.

Marshmallow Root 1:5 Glycetract (MediHerb): Provides demulcent activity which is useful for irritations of the oral and pharyngeal mucosa, dry cough, and chronic irritable cough.

Dosage: Three mL, once to twice per day.

Candidiasis

Defined

Candidiasis is an infection with, or disease caused by, *Candida,* especially *Candida albicans.*

Candida albicans is a normal inhabitant of the gastrointestinal tract, skin, mouth, and vaginal canal. Candida overgrowth results in a wide variety of localized and systemic symptoms. The most common areas affected are the skin, oral mucous membranes (thrush), esophagus (esophagitis), respiratory tract (pulmonary Candidiasis), vagina (vaginal yeast infection), and gastrointestinal tract. Systemic infections can be the result of a compromised immune system, or the result of yeast cells, particles of yeast cells, or toxins from yeast "die off" entering the systemic circulation as a result of a disruption of the intestinal lining (leaky gut). Systemic candidiasis can have an affect on the heart, brain, and nervous, immune, genitourinary, and endocrine systems. Candidiasis can be more severe in immunocompromised patients.

Signs and Symptoms

These are some of the more common complaints regarding Candidiasis.

- Fatigue
- Intestinal bloating, gas
- Constipation or diarrhea
- Premenstrual syndrome
- Depression, anxiety
- Difficulty concentrating

- Recurrent bladder infections
- Vaginal itch and burning
- Food allergies
- Sensitivity to smells
- Sugar (refined carbohydrate) cravings

Etiology

- Poor liver function
- Weakened immunity
- Poor digestive functioning
- Systemic use of antibacterial, immunosuppressive, and corticosteroid therapy
- Diet high in dairy products (e.g. processed pasteurized milk and cheese)
- Endocrinopathies

- Bowel flora imbalance
- High sugar intake
- Obesity
- Diabetes mellitus
- Nutrient deficiency
- Chronic illness
- Use of birth control pills

Symptoms

These are some of the more common complaints regarding Candidiasis.

- Fatigue
- Intestinal bloating, gas
- Constipation or diarrhea
- Premenstrual syndrome
- Depression, anxiety
- Difficulty concentrating

- Recurrent bladder infections
- Vaginal itch and burning
- Food allergies
- Sensitivity to smells
- Sugar (refined carbohydrate) cravings

Candidiasis

Treatment Considerations

- Digestion plays a central role in the prevention of Candidiasis. Therefore, particular attention should be paid to such remedies that aid digestion such as betaine hydrochloride, pancreatic enzymes, and remedies that support bile production and flow.
- Reduce stool pH to create an environment that is not conducive to Candida overgrowth.
- Use anti-fungal and anti-microbial remedies.
- Support overall immune functioning. Recurrent or chronic Candidiasis will, over time, result in a compromised immune system.
- Enhance liver detoxification mechanisms. If food and chemical sensitivities are issues, liver support is essential.
- Re-establish healthy intestinal microflora with the use of probiotics.

Supplementation

Primary Support

Zymex® (Capsules) (Standard Process): Specialized yeast culture that supports the formation of lactic acid from carbohydrates in the large intestine, which results in lowering the pH of the stool. This effect promotes a healthy balance of intestinal flora and creates an environment which is not conducive to *Candida albicans* overgrowth.

Dosage: Two to three capsules, three times per day with meals.

Note: Zymex® contains lactose. With patients who may have an issue with this, recommend Lactic Acid Yeast™ (Standard Process) instead of Zymex®. These are in a wafer form with the dosage being two-three wafers three times per day with meals.

Garlic 5000mg (MediHerb): Garlic has antifungal and anti-parasitic qualities. The enteric coating on the tablets ensures maximum delivery of the various sulfur containing compounds to the small and large intestine. It is these sulfur containing compounds that provide the antifungal and antiparasitic actions.

Dosage: One tablet, three times per day with or without meals.

Spanish Black Radish (Standard Process): A very good source of sulfur. Sulfur is beneficial for the healthy functioning of the enterocytes lining the gastrointestinal tract.

Dosage: Two tablets, three times per day with meals.

Cat's Claw Complex (MediHerb): The combined action of Cat's Claw, Pau d'Arco, and Echinacea provide antifungal, antiparasitic, and immune enhancing actions.

Dosage: One tablet, three to four times per day with or without food.

LactEnz® (Standard Process):. It is a source of *Lactobacillus acidophilus* and *Bifidobacterium longum* along with protease, amylase, lipase, and cellulase. Start Lact-Enz® approximately one month after beginning Zymex® (Capsules), Spanish Black Radish, Garlic 5000mg, and Cat's Claw Complex. Introduce this probiotic only after the environment is conducive to accept the probiotic.

Dosage: Three capsules, two times per day at least one hour before or two hours after a meal is preferred. Taking the capsules on an empty stomach maximizes delivery of the probiotic into the small and large intestine.

Use this protocol for twelve weeks along with the lifestyle recommendations noted below.

Note: Digestive dysfunction is common for patients with Candidiasis. Refer to the section titled *Inadequate Digestion* for further information.

Secondary Support: As Indicated

Golden Seal 500mg (MediHerb): A berberine-containing herb noted for its broad-spectrum antifungal and antibacterial qualities. It is useful, in this respect, for intestinal support but additionally for its mucous membrane trophorestorative properties.

Dosage: One tablet, three times per day.

Immuplex® (Standard Process): Provides the vitamin A, C, and E complexes, folic acid, cyanocobalamin, trace minerals, liver, thymus, spleen, and bone Protomorphogen™ extracts along with other synergistic factors for optimal immune system support. This is a product to be considered for depleted immune systems that require specific nutritional factors to optimize the immune response.

Dosage: Two capsules, three times per day with meals.

Note: To support liver detoxification pathways, refer to the section titled *Detoxification*.

Lifestyle Recommendations

Due to the high rate of relapse among people with Candida overgrowth, the following lifestyle modifications are recommended during the 12-week supplement protocol:

- For optimal results, the patient should remove all dairy products and refined sugars from the diet during the twelve weeks.
- Avoid alcoholic beverages.
- Avoid foods with high mold/fungal content. Some examples being dried fruits, peanuts, and fermented products, such as cheeses and vinegar.

Cardiac Arrhythmias

Defined

Any abnormality in the regularity, rate, or sequence of cardiac activation. Arrhythmias vary in severity – from mild, asymptomatic, and requiring no treatment (such as sinus arrhythmia, in which the heart rate increases and decreases with respiration) to severe ventricular fibrillation, which required resuscitation. Arrhythmias are generally classified according to their origin (supraventricular or ventricular). Their effect on blood pressure and cardiac output, partially influenced by the site of origin, determines their clinical significance. (Refer to the appropriate texts for more information regarding the various types of cardiac arrhythmias.)

Signs and Symptoms

Symptoms of arrhythmias result from reduced cardiac output and altered perfusion to the organs and may include:

- Dyspnea
- Asymptomatic
- Dizziness, syncope, and weakness
- Hypotension
- Chest pain
- Cool, clammy skin
- Altered level of consciousness
- Palpitations
- Reduced urinary output

Etiology

Each arrhythmia can have its own specific causes. Common causes include:

- Myocardial infarction or ischemia
- Congenital defects
- Drug toxicity
- Organic heart disease
- Connective tissue disorders
- Obstruction or degeneration of conductive tissue
- Electrolyte imbalances
- Acid-base imbalances
- Emotional stress
- Hypertrophy of the heart muscle
- Digestive toxins carried to the heart from the lymphatic system
- Nutritional status, especially the concentration of B vitamin components and mineral content as this could alter the sodium-potassium pump, depolarization, and refractory period of nerve fibers

Treatment Considerations

- Provide those nutrients needed for optimal nerve conductivity and ATP production
- Improve oxygenation and nutrient delivery to the heart

Cardia Arrhythmias

Supplementation

Primary Support

Vasculin® (Standard Process): Provides the following:

- Cataplex® B: Source of B vitamin components and naturally occurring associated factors that are needed for optimal cardiac electrical activity as well as ATP production. The thiamine in Cataplex® B reduces lactic acid buildup which is important in an oxygen starved heart
- Heart Protomorphogen™ extract.
- Cataplex® E: Source of the vitamin E complex and synergistic cofactors which together provide antioxidant protection and connective tissue repair factors, also supports oxygen delivery to cardiac tissue.
- Connective tissue Protomorphogen™ extracts: Support for the fibrous strands (chordae tendinae) running from the papillary muscles to the leaflets of the atrioventricular valves.

Dosage: Two capsules, three times per day with meals.

Cardio-Plus® (Standard Process): Provides the following:

- Cataplex® C: Vitamin C components enhance the blood's oxygen carrying capacity, support adrenal gland functioning, and provide antioxidant protection.
- Adrenal Cytosol™ extract: Optimal adrenal functioning is essential since these glands do back up cardiac functioning. For example; the adrenal glands offer indirect cardiac support by providing the epinephrine push that occurs when one goes from a supine to an upright position.
- Cataplex® G: Provides B vitamins, which have a dilatory effect on coronary arteries.
- Heart Protomorphogen™ extract.

Dosage: Three tablets, three times per day with meals.

Hawthorn (MediHerb): Hawthorn provides cardiotonic, cardioprotective, hypotensive, antiarrhythmic, antioxidant, and vasodilatory actions.

Dosage: One tablet, three times per day.

Secondary Support: As Indicated

Calcium Lactate (Standard Process): Source of ionizable calcium to ensure optimal release of acetylcholine from synaptic vesicles at the neuromuscular junction.

Dosage: Three to four tablets, three times per day. Best taken between meals.

Organically Bound Minerals (Standard Process): Source of potassium which is necessary for normal nerve depolarization.

Dosage: One tablet, three times per day with meals.

Cirrhosis - Hepatic

Defined

Cirrhosis is damage or death of liver cells resulting in the formation of diffuse interlacing fibrotic tissue.

Signs and Symptoms

Early stage cirrhosis:

- Nausea and vomiting; diarrhea; anorexia
- Dull abdominal ache

Late stage cirrhosis:

- Endocrine: menstrual irregularities, testicular atrophy, loss of chest hair and axillary hair, gynecomastia
- Hematologic: splenomegaly, anemia, bleeding tendency, portal hypertension
- Respiratory: limited thoracic expansion, pleural effusion, impaired gas exchange
- Central nervous system: progressive signs and symptoms of hepatic encephalopathy, including extreme obtundation, coma, lethargy
- Skin: extreme dryness and poor tissue turgor, severe pruritis, palmar erythema, spider angiomas
- Hepatic: hepatomegaly, jaundice, edema and ascites of the legs, hepatorenal syndrome
- Miscellaneous: enlarged superficial abdominal veins, musty breath, temperature of 101° to 103° (38° to 39° C), pain in the right upper abdominal quadrant when the patient leans forward or sits up

Etiology

Cholestatic diseases:

- Biliary cirrhosis: prolonged obstruction of the bile duct, inflammation

Metabolic diseases:

- Wilson's disease
- Alpha-1antitrypsin deficiency
- Hemochromatosis

Hepatocellular diseases:

- Post necrotic cirrhosis: toxic exposure, viral hepatitis
- Autoimmune disease, such as chronic inflammatory bowel disease or sarcoidosis
- Portal, nutritional, or alcoholic cirrhosis

Other:

- Cardiac cirrhosis: right sided heart failure
- Budd-Chiari syndrome: obstruction of the hepatic vein
- Cryptogenic cirrhosis: unknown etiology

Treatment Considerations

- Nutritional support to ensure optimal hepatocellular functioning
- Hepatoprotective and trophorestorative support
- Antioxidants to protect and maintain the hepatocytes

Cirrhosis - Hepatic

Supplementation

Primary Support: First 30 Days

Silymarin (MediHerb): Hepatoprotective and hepatotrophorestorative support.

Dosage: Two tablets, twice per day.

Hepatrophin PMG® (Standard Process): Liver Protomorphogen™ extract support.

Dosage: Two tablets, three times per day with meals.

Cataplex® G (Standard Process): Provides lipotrophic factors and B vitamin components with the greatest affinity for supporting liver restoration.

Dosage: Two tablets, three times per day with meals.

Primary Support: After 30 Days

Silymarin (MediHerb): Hepatoprotective and hepatotrophorestorative support.

Dosage: Two tablets, twice per day.

OPC Synergy™ (Standard Process): Broad antioxidant support provided by green tea extract, grape seed extract, red wine extract, bilberry, carrot powder, and buckwheat juice powder.

Dosage: One capsule, two to three times per day with meals.

Hepatrophin PMG® (Standard Process): Liver Protomorphogen™ extract support.

Dosage: Two tablets, three times per day with meals.

Livaplex® (Standard Process): This formula is a combination of ingredients which support the following actions: bile production and flow, bowel detoxification, liver decongestion (due to lipotrophic factors), hepatic Protomorphogen™ extract support, and enhanced blood flow through the portal vein.

Dosage: Two to three capsules, three times per day with meals.

Super-Eff® (Standard Process): The liver is responsible for the degradation of fatty acids into small compounds that can be used for energy and to synthesize other lipids from fatty acids, specifically cholesterol and phospholipids. The liver is also one of the largest "consumers" of fatty acids in the body. Supper-Eff is a source of pre-processed fatty acids after they have been metabolized by the liver.

Dosage: Two tablets, three times per day with meals.

Chlorophyll Complex™ (Standard Process): Chlorophyll is an excellent source of the fat-soluble vitamins of which the liver has a high affinity for.

Dosage: One to two perles, three times per day with meals.

Note: For additional nutritional support regarding the liver, refer to the section titled *General Liver Support.*

Common Cold & Flu (Acute Rhinitis)

Defined

A catarrhal disorder of the upper respiratory tract which can be bacterial, viral, a mixed infection, or an allergic reaction that causes inflammation of the upper respiratory tract.

Signs and Symptoms

- Pharyngitis
- Fever
- Coryza
- Lethargy
- Chills
- Myalgia
- Arthralgia
- Headache
- Sore throat
- Clear watery discharge followed by mucopurulent discharge
- Sequalae can include sinusitis, otitis media, and tonsillitis

Etiology

The majority of colds are from a viral infection of the upper respiratory passages and consequent mucous membrane inflammation; colds can occasionally result from a mycoplasmal infection. Many viruses can cause the common cold. Major offenders include:

- Coronaviruses
- Rhinoviruses
- Adenoviruses
- Coxsackieviruses
- Myxoviruses
- Echoviruses

Treatment Considerations

- Enhance immune function with nutritional supplementation and herbal remedies.
- Use diaphoretics to promote sweating and thereby help modulate a fever.
- Employ mucolytic and anticatarrhal agents.
- Make use of antiviral herbs when appropriate.
- Encourage fluid intake to prevent dehydration.

Supplementation

Primary Support

Andrographis Complex (MediHerb): This formula is immune enhancing and immune modulating, consider for any upper respiratory conditions when the previously noted actions are desired.

Dosage: Two tablets, four times per day until the bottle is finished.

Common Cold & Flu (Acute Rhinitis)

Cal-Amo® (Standard Process): This is an acidifying compound which helps to maintain the proper pH balance at the cellular level. A proper acid/alkaline balance is necessary to maintain healthy respiratory tissues as well as supporting the immune system.

Dosage: Two tablets, three times per day with meals until the bottle is finished.

Congaplex® (Standard Process): Congaplex® is a combination of the vitamin C and A complexes, thymus Cytosol™ extract, calcium lactate, and cellular protein precursor material in the form of ribonucleic acid. This formula provides the nutrients the immune system requires to mount an efficient immune response.

Dosage: Adult: Four to six capsules, three times per day with meals until the bottle is finished.
       Child: Two capsules, three times per day with meals until the bottle is finished

DiaCo Phytosynergist™ (MediHerb): Diaphoretic formula. This product is only to be used if fever is present.

- Anti-infective
- Immunostimulant
- Diaphoretic
- Anticatarrhal
- Mucolytic
- Expectorant

Dosage: Five mL, three to five times per day with a small glass of warm water until fever subsides, then discontinue. Can be sipped as a tea.

Secondary Support: As Indicated

Echinacea Premium (MediHerb): To enhance the immune response.

Dosage: One tablet, three times per day for additional immune support.

St. John's Wort 1.8g (MediHerb): Antiviral, specific against enveloped viruses, St. John's Wort is a useful adjunct with influenza A & B.

Dosage: One tablet, three to four times per day.

Constipation

Defined

Difficult or infrequent bowel movements. Constipation also refers to hardness of stool or a feeling of incomplete evacuation.

Signs and Symptoms

- Stools may be small, hard, and difficult to expel
- Regular use of laxatives
- Nausea
- Halitosis
- Excessive flatulence
- Abdominal bloating after eating

Etiology

- Low fluid intake
- Low fiber diet
- Lack of exercise
- Age
- Inadequate bile production and flow (poor liver function)
- Drugs
- Low thyroid function
- Irritable bowel syndrome
- Insufficient production of hydrolyzing digestive enzymes
- Congenital megacolon
- Multiple sclerosis, Muscular Dystrophy
- Trauma
- Scleroderma
- Rectal or colonic carcinoma
- Diverticulosis
- Chronic laxative use
- Pregnancy
- Intestinal fungal overgrowth
- Parasitic infestation
- Anxiety, stress, depression
- Bowel flora imbalance
- Pituitary disorders

Treatment Considerations

- Constipation can be a symptom of another underlying health issue. If constipation of recent onset persists, or if a patient with chronic constipation has never been fully evaluated, a more thorough investigation is needed to determine the cause of constipation.
- Although effective in promoting peristalsis, the use of stimulant laxatives should be limited.
- Natural approaches aimed at improving hepatic production and flow of bile, along with bulking agents, lubricating agents, foods, and herbs that improve bowel function should be considered.

Supplementation

Primary Support: Stimulating Bowel Elimination

To stimulate bowel elimination, <u>choose one</u> of the following three products.

Colax (MediHerb): A gentle formula supporting increased bile flow and production while simultaneously promoting regular intestinal elimination through anthraquinone-containing herbs.

Dosage: Start with two tablets before bed and allow a few days to determine the status of elimination. It is important to increase water intake while taking this formula. If two tablets do not address the issues adequately, increase to four tablets at bedtime. The dosage can be increased up to six before bed if needed. It is recommended that Colax not be used indefinitely. If the product is used for six weeks, a two to three week hiatus should be taken before resuming.

Clinical Note: If Colax does not promote regular elimination, this indicates an imbalance in the intestinal microflora. The beneficial bacteria needed to cleave off a sugar molecule from the anthraquinones are not present in a dysbiotic gut. This process is necessary in order to create the laxative effect. Refer to the sections titled *Bowel Dysbiosis* and/or *Candidiasis* if Colax is ineffective.

Constipation

Fen-Cho® (Standard Process): The combination of bile salts, Collinsonia root, and fenugreek seed make this an effective stool softener with a gentle laxative effect. Use this product when hard dry stools are evident. For these situations recommend the patient drink six to eight glasses of water per day to ensure adequate hydration.

Dosage: Begin with two tablets in the morning and allow a day or two to pass to see if this is enough to promote peristalsis. Increase the dosage to two tablets twice per day and up to two tablets three times per day with a <u>full glass</u> of water as the case dictates. Maximum dosage is three to four tablets three times per day with a glass of water.

Gastro-Fiber® (Standard Process): The combination of psyllium husk powder, Collinsonia root powder, apple pectin, fennel seed, and fenugreek seed powder provide the mucilaginous material, fiber, gas dispelling, smooth muscle relaxant, and peristaltic promotion qualities needed in a gentle fiber formula. Good adjunct when the diet is low in fiber.

Dosage: Two capsules before bed and two capsules upon arising initially and increase up to two capsules three times per day if needed. Ensure adequate water intake while on this formula.

Primary Support: Utilization of Choleretics and Cholagogues

A recommended approach would be to utilize one Standard Process and one Mediherb product together. This will provide optimal nutrient delivery to support the production and flow of bile, a natural laxative, while at the same time employing the use of herbs to support healthy liver and gallbladder functioning.

A-F Betafood® (Standard Process): Provides those nutrients needed to ensure optimal hepatic production of bile. This product is a good source of betaine, from red beets, which has a thinning effect on the bile. Also contains lipotrophic agents which promote the transportation and use of fats, thus helping to prevent the accumulation of fat in the liver.

Dosage: Two to three tablets, three times per day with meals. For difficult cases, consider up to five tablets three times per day with meals for two weeks and then reduce the dosage accordingly.

Betafood® (Standard Process): This product mainly consists of beet root and beet greens thus containing higher amounts of the bile thinning factors than A-F Betafood®.

Dosage: Two to three tablets, three times per day with meals.

Livaplex® (Standard Process): This formula is a combination of six individual Standard Process products. In addition to supporting bile production and flow, this product also supports bowel detoxification and liver decongestion due to the lipotrophic factors, provides hepatic Protomorphogen™ extract support, and provides for enhanced blood flow through the portal vein.

Dosage: Two to three capsules, three times per day with food.

Livton® Complex (MediHerb): The combination of Greater Celandine, Milk Thistle, Fringe Tree, and Globe Artichoke make this an herbal remedy in tablet form that supports bile production and flow.

Dosage: One tablet, three times a day with meals.

Globe Artichoke 1:2 (MediHerb): Bitter tonic, choleretic, and cholagogue.

Dosage: Two mL, twice a day.

Clinical Notes

Patients with constipation are advised to make the following lifestyle modifications:

- The diet should contain sufficient amounts of fiber to ensure adequate stool bulk. Vegetables and fruits are recommended.
- Drink adequate water. Dehydration is an often overlooked cause of constipation.
- Include healthy fats, such as flaxseed oil and extra virgin olive oil, etc., as a regular part of the diet; avoid margarine and other hydrogenated fats.
- Replace coffee with herbal teas, such as chamomile or roasted Dandelion root.

Bladder Infection (Cystitis)

Defined

Inflammation of the urinary bladder.

Signs and Symptoms

- Frequency, urgency, dysuria
- Nocturia
- Hematuria
- Chills, fever
- Itching and/or a feeling of warmth during urination
- Flank pain, low back pain
- Abdominal pain, tenderness over the bladder area
- Malaise

Etiology

- Bacteria ascending from a colonized vaginal and urethra to the bladder
- Intestinal bacteria could be an etiological factor regarding bladder infections due to the close proximity of the anal area to the urethra
- Infections can be derived from the blood
- Incomplete emptying of the bladder due to lack of muscular tone
- Sexual intercourse
- Catheterization
- Pregnant women have twice the frequency of cystitis
- In men, the most common etiological factor regarding recurring cystitis is a persistent bacterial infection of the prostate, however an ascending infection of the urethra could also be a factor
- Compromised urine flow (e.g. kidney stone, enlarged prostate)
- Excess sugar consumption
- Can be a sequalae of Candida albicans proliferation
- Breakdown of local defense mechanisms in the bladder that allow bacteria to invade the bladder mucosa and multiply

Note: Untreated, chronic urinary tract infections can eventually lead to infection of the kidneys.

Treatment Considerations

Herbal and nutritional support in uncomplicated cystitis cases can be very effective. However, one should always keep in mind that pyelonephritis (kidney infection) can be a sequel to cystitis. If a fever should develop with or without back pain in addition to any other symptoms, referral for allopathic treatment may be required.

Desired actions of suggested remedies:

- Urinary tract antiseptics
- Demulcents
- Diuretics
- Immune stimulation
- Reduce adherence of bacteria to bladder wall
- Promote optimal pH of urine to inhibit bacterial growth in the bladder
- Nutritional support to enhance local tissue integrity

Bladder Infection (Cystitis)

Supplementation

Primary Support

Cal-Amo® (Standard Process): Provides the acidifying compounds that are useful in maintaining the proper acid/alkaline balance.

Dosage: Two tablets, three times per day with meals. Finish the entire bottle.

Congaplex® (Standard Process): This is to be used during the acute phase. The combination of the vitamin C and A complexes, thymus Cytosol™ extract, calcium lactate, and cellular protein precursor material in the form of RNA, provide the immune system the nutrients required in order to mount an efficient immune response.

Dosage: Four to six capsules, three times per day with meals. Finish the entire bottle.

UriCo Phytosynergist™ (MediHerb):

- Provides a urinary antiseptic
- Soothes the mucous membranes
- Decreases the pain and frequency of urination
- Enhances the immune response

Dosage: Five mL, four to five times per day until the bottle is finished.

Clinical Note: Use one bottle of the UriCo Phytosynergist™. For an acute condition, consider adding MediHerb's Andrographis Complex (six/day) in conjunction with the UriCo Phytosynergist™. If the history reveals recurrent UTI's, follow up with MediHerb's Cranberry Complex (see below) long term after finishing the UriCo Phytosynergist™.

During the acute phase, patients should be drinking sufficient quantities of water and avoiding coffee, alcohol, soft drinks, and juices. Refined carbohydrates and simple sugars should be avoided entirely.

Secondary Support: As Indicated

Cranberry Complex (MediHerb): Urinary antiseptic and muscular tonic for the bladder for recurrent urinary tract infections (can also be used instead of the UriCo Phytosynergist™).

Dosage: One tablet, three times per day long term or two tablets three times per day for acute cases. Can be used prophylactically after the acute episode.

Cataplex® A-C (Standard Process): Provides the vitamin A and C complex factors to support the immune system as well as the maintenance of healthy epithelial and connective tissues.

Dosage: Two tablets, three times per day with meals.

Golden Seal 500mg (MediHerb): With anti-microbial and mucous membrane trophorestorative properties, Golden Seal 500mg is useful in healing an inflamed and irritated bladder epithelium.

Dosage: One tablet, three times per day.

Depression (Mild to Moderate)

Defined

Depression is a mental state of depressed mood characterized by feelings of despair, sadness, and discouragement. The ranges of depression are from normal feelings of the blues through dysthmia to major depression. Dysthmia is characterized by depressed feelings (such as sad, blue, low, down in the dumps, and loss of interest in one's usual activities) that have persisted for more than two years and are not severe enough to meet the criteria for major depression.

A person must have five or more of the symptoms listed below occurring on a regular basis for at least two years before an official diagnosis of clinical depression can be made. For additional information on depression, refer to the Diagnostic and Statistical Manual of Mental Disorders (DSM-IV).

Symptoms

- Poor appetite
- Increased appetite
- Insomnia
- Excessive sleeping
- Hyperactivity
- Fatigue and/or weakness
- Decreased activity
- Can't complete tasks
- Withdrawal from society
- Headaches, backaches, & digestive disorders

- Chronic nervousness
- Decreased libido
- Quickness to anger
- Low self esteem
- Difficulty concentrating
- Thoughts of suicide
- Increased susceptibility to infections

The presence of five or more of the above may indicate depression.

Treatment Considerations

In practice, we often see mild to moderate depression brought about by nutritional deficiency and/or stress in the patient's life. This stress can be an emotional event, relationship issues, and/or ill health. The use of nutritional and herbal remedies can be effective for mild to moderate depression, and can be especially useful during tumultuous events.

There are times when we need to recommend more than just an antidepressant remedy. Consideration of other conditions or pathologies should also be addressed because these can cause or contribute to depression. For example: depression can be caused by adrenal fatigue, thyroid disorders, chronic pain, hormonal imbalances, and nutritional deficiencies.

Note: Episodes of major (clinical) depression should be referred to a psychotherapist or psychiatrist for appropriate treatment.

Supplementation
Primary Support

Min-Chex® (Standard Process): Contains calcium, magnesium, kelp, Niacinamide B6, orchic Cytosol™ extract along with those nutrients that function synergistically to support the parasympathetic nervous system and enhance oxygen delivery to the brain.

Dosage: Two capsules three times per day with meals.

Depression (Mild to Moderate)

Note: An excellent alternative to Min-Chex® is Min-Tran® (Standard Process). Min-Tran® is chiefly composed of calcium lactate, magnesium, kelp and alfalfa. It is higher in calcium and magnesium that Min-Chex®, but does not contain the orchic Cytosol™ extract or Niacinamide B6. Min-Tran® could be considered a mineral tranquilizer.

Dosage: Three to four tablets three times per day with meals.

Protefood® (Standard Process): Source of essential and heat labile amino acids. People today can be sub-clinically vitamin deficient due to certain cofactors missing in the diet. For example, dietary tryptophan can be converted to nicotinamide in the body. Since tryptophan is a heat labile amino acid, a lack of this amino acid could result in dementia.

Dosage: One tablet three times per day with meals.

Note: For a complete amino acid supplement, consider Nutrimere® (Standard Process) at a dosage of one capsule three times per day with meals in place of Protefood®.

Cataplex® G (Standard Process): Source of B vitamins and synergistic factors that support the parasympathetic nervous system thus acting as a calmative.

Dosage: Two tablets three times per day with meals.

St John's Wort 1.8g (MediHerb): Appropriate for mild to moderate depression.

Dosage: Three to four tablets per day.

Secondary Support: As Indicated

Nevaton® (MediHerb): Combines the actions of St. John's Wort, Damiana, Skullcap, and Schisandra to support patients who are depressed and suffering from anxiety. This formula can be combined successfully with Valerian Complex (MediHerb).

Dosage: One tablet three to four times per day if used alone.

Note: If used in conjunction with St John's Wort 1.8g, then reduce the St John's Wort 1.8g tablets to one tablet twice per day.

Valerian Complex (MediHerb): Support for those dealing with stress and anxiety through the combined actions of Spiny jujube, Valerian, and Passionflower.

Dosage: Three to four tablets per day.

With any emotional issues, the resulting increase in sympathetic response puts tremendous strain on the adrenal glands. Couple this with a poor or inadequate diet and one can see why those individuals suffering from depression and/or anxiety for example may and in all likelihood need adrenal support. Refer to the sections titled Adrenal Fatigue and/ or Hypothyroidism for additional information on topics related to depression.

Detoxification

Detoxification (also known as internal cleansing or purification) has been in use for over a century. The issue of toxicity has arisen because of our increasing exposure to toxins in our water, air, and food. Simply couple this with a poor diet that does not support optimal cellular functioning, and the impact upon health can become devastating.

The body removes toxins by direct filtration in the liver or by excreting those toxins as part of the bile or urine after the toxins have been processed by the liver. The mechanism by which the liver processes the toxins is the cytochrome P450 phase I and phase II pathways. Toxins are also removed via the cytochrome P450 phase I enzyme system in the lungs, brain, kidneys, adrenal cortex, testes, spleen, heart, muscles, skin, and in the cells lining the intestine.

The liver has many roles in detoxification. It filters the blood, produces and secretes bile, and enzymatically processes toxic chemicals. The process of detoxification and the preparation of the toxins for excretion take place in two distinct biochemical phases, known as the cytochrome P450 phase I and phase II detoxification pathways. Phase I can either convert the toxin to a water soluble form to be excreted either through the bile or urine, or modify the toxin to what is referred to as a primary metabolite. Primary metabolites are acted upon by one or more of the several phase II processes. In Phase II, the conjugating substances are attached to the phase I product (primary metabolite) to facilitate its excretion through the bile or urine. Phase II reactions typically take place through methylation, glucuronidaton, acetylation, sulfation, glutathione conjugation and amino acid conjugation. If the phase I-generated reactive molecules (primary metabolite) are not transformed into excretable compounds, toxic intermediates can build up.

Weight Management

The National Institutes of Health (NIH); the National Heart, Lung, and Blood Institute (NHLBI); the National Health and Nutrition Examination Survey (NHANES); leading medical journals; and the media all report that many Americans are overweight. How is this happening? Americans are consuming large portions of the wrong kinds of foods, such as refined foods and snacks high in sugar, instead of balanced meals that include good-quality proteins (fresh meat, poultry, and fish), fruits, vegetables, and small amounts of whole grains. These poor diet choices combined with a sedentary lifestyle promote weight gain.

Many Americans address their weight issues by trying quick-fix weight management programs. Because these programs do not take into account the long term needs of the body, these dieters do not experience permanent results. In addition, many quick-fix programs are not designed to be utilized for an extended period of time. Post-dieters who go on these programs become frustrated because eventually all the weight that was lost comes back.

The ideal weight management program does take time. It needs to be gentle, reduce excess fat stores, be high in fiber and lower in fat, and ensure that the amount of metabolic energy being used is greater than the amount of calories consumed. Once the ideal weight is reached, maintaining it requires that the amount of energy expended is equal to the energy intake.

Our bodies are like cars with a main fuel tank and a reserve tank. When one tank runs dry, the engine draws fuel from the reserve tank to meet its needs. Our bodies run in a similar fashion. Say for instance, a person walks on a treadmill for 20-30 minutes. During this time, they have burned off their main fuel – the sugar in their blood, liver, and muscles. Once that fuel is depleted, their body turns to fat (their reserve fuel tank) for additional energy.

Healthy liver function supports the body in burning fat for energy. The nutrients and dietary recommendations in the Standard Process purification program revolve around feeding the body the nutrients it needs to support optimal liver function. In addition to its role in fat burning, the liver also synthesizes fatty acids from amino acids and sugars and assists in producing lipoproteins, cholesterol, and phospholipids. The liver manufacturers the glucose tolerance factor (GTF) from chromium and glutathione. GTF partners with the body's natural insulin to regulate and maintain healthy blood sugar levels. The liver converts any sugars that are not required for immediate energy needs into glycogen, cholesterol, and fat. Glycogen is stored both in the liver and in muscle tissue. The fat and cholesterol can be deposited in areas such as the buttocks, abdominal region and vasculature.

Detoxification

The Standard Process purification program is a gentle program that feeds the body, more specifically the liver, the nutrients it needs so it can perform the actions normally required of it. At the same time, the program requires that the patient make lifestyle changes to aid in the removal of the majority of toxins they are exposed to and modify the diet to stabilize insulin levels.

Note: The Standard Process purification program is remarkably effective when your patients follow the instructions as put forth in the Patient Guide. This guide goes into more detail about how to implement the program. You can obtain this booklet from your Standard Process representative/distributor or through the Standard Process Home Office. It is suggested that you obtain these booklets and any associated material pertaining to the program before instituting the purification program in a clinical setting.

Purification Products

The following Standard Process products are used as important components of the purification program: SP Cleanse®, SP Complete™, Gastro-Fiber®, and SP Green Food™.

SP Cleanse®

SP Cleanse enlists the detoxifying properties of over 20 different whole foods and botanicals in this vegetarian nutritional supplement. The phytonutrients from these ingredients help the body eliminate exogenous toxins along with the end products of cellular metabolism.

The vitamin complexes, minerals, and phytonutrients in SP Cleanse support the body's elimination routes by:

- Maintaining healthy liver detoxification function
- Encouraging healthy kidney function
- Promoting efficient gastrointestinal elimination
- Supporting lymphatic system function
- Helping to maintain healthy blood

SP Complete™

SP Complete is a whole food and botanical supplement that can be blended with water and fruit to make a nutritious supplement shake. It offers a balance of essential macro- and micronutrients from plant sources in a highly bioavailable form.

The natural whole food ingredients used to formulate SP Complete deliver powerful antioxidant components that promote cellular health and support healthy cardiovascular, digestive, and nervous system function. Whether taken alone or with meals, a supplement shake made with SP Complete provides essential vitamins and minerals during the purification process.

Gastro-Fiber®

Dietary fiber comes from the cellular walls of plants and has specific effects on different aspects of gastrointestinal function. Gastro-Fiber contains phytonutrients from psyllium, Collinsonia root, apple pectin, fennel seed, and fenugreek seed. These whole-food factors function synergistically to:

- Help cleanse and lubricate the intestines
- Encourage regular elimination
- Promote pH balance throughout the gastrointestinal tract
- Supports short chain fatty acid production

SP Green Food™

SP Green Food is made up of five organically grown whole food concentrates: Brussels sprouts, kale, alfalfa, buckwheat, and barley grass. In addition to their natural bioavailability, these foods contain vitamins, minerals, and other unknown synergistic cofactors that support the cytochrome P450 phase I and phase II detoxification pathways.

Program Choices

There are two programs from which to recommend: Optimal Intensity Program and Modified Intensity Program. Both will offer many benefits to your patients. Choose the one that best fits your patient's particular needs.

Detoxification

Note: If your patient does not have a weight issue, you may want to consider implementing the Modified Intensity Program. If there are blood sugar issues, such as Type I or Type II diabetes, then these programs may have to be modified in order to meet the specific needs of the individual.

Optimal Intensity Program: Garden Variety

Garden Variety is a purification program that consists of eating only vegetables and fruits. Vegetables contain many vital nutrients, and their enzymes work as natural cleansing agents. Raw vegetables have stronger cleansing ability than cooked, but all vegetables are beneficial. For example; beets purify the blood; asparagus promotes healthy kidney function; and artichokes enhance liver function.

Food Intake: Weeks 1-3

For the first three weeks, patients should consume only the items listed here in addition to their supplements and shakes. Use organic fruits and vegetables if available.

- **Unlimited fresh vegetables**

  - Collard greens*
  - Dandelion greens
  - Mixed greens
  - Mustard greens
  - Red, yellow, and green peppers
  - Onions*
  - Mushrooms
  - Spinach
  - Carrots

  - Radishes
  - Kale*
  - Broccoli*
  - Swiss chard*
  - Brussels sprouts*
  - Asparagus*
  - Cabbage*
  - Cucumbers
  - Celery
  - Red beets (Beets may be steamed for 20-30 minutes or until soft. Patients may use the beet greens in salads after washing.)

  *May be steamed for four minutes

- **Salads with unlimited fresh vegetables**

  - Salad dressings are **not** permissible
  - Nuts, seeds, and beans (including green beans) are **not** permissible

- **Fruit – eat twice as many vegetables as compared to fruit (1 serving = 1 cup)**

  - Examples include but are not limited to:

• Apples	• Berries
• Oranges	• Melons
• Bananas	• Tomatoes
• Grapes	

    Avocadoes are not permissible

- **Spring water (at least 8 glasses per day)**

REFRAIN FROM HAVING THE PATIENT CONSUME ANYTHING NOT LISTED
When followed as directed, this purification program has shown in clinical practice to offer great rewards in terms of desired outcomes and patient satisfaction. Any alteration of the instructions allows for variables that could decrease the benefits of the program; therefore, it is recommended that the instructions are followed completely and not modified.

Supplementation – Garden Variety

SP Complete™ and Gastro-Fiber® are recommended throughout the Garden Variety program; SP Cleanse® is recommended for week one only; and SP Green Food™ is recommended for weeks two and three.

Detoxification

Week One
- 2-3 SP Complete shakes per day
  (refer to the last page of this section for the shake recipe)
- 7 SP Cleanse capsules 3 times daily without food/but with shakes or water
- 3 Gastro-Fiber capsules 3 times daily without food/but with shakes or water

Weeks Two & Three
- 2-3 SP Complete shakes per day
- 3 Gastro-Fiber capsules 3 times daily without food/but with shakes or water
- 5 SP Green Food capsules 2 times daily without food/but with shakes or water

> **PLEASE NOTE THAT SUPPLEMENTS SHOULD BE TAKEN WITH A SP COMPLETE SHAKE OR WATER, BUT NOT WITH FOOD. THE SUPPLEMENTS MAY ALSO BE TAKEN RIGHT BEFORE BED.**

Exercise
It is recommended that the patients walk at least 4 times per week for 30-45 minutes. Strenuous exercise should be avoided during the three-week period.

Modified Intensity Program: Wholesome Medley

Wholesome medley is a purification program that consists of eating vegetables, fruits, and protein. The whole foods in Wholesome Medley support all the major organ systems during purification.

Food Intake: Weeks 1-3
For the first three weeks, only the items listed below should be consumed in addition to the supplements and shakes. Use organic fruits and vegetables if available.

- **3-4 oz. of unseasoned meat, fish, or poultry twice daily**
  Simply prepared – broiling, baking, etc.

- **Unlimited fresh vegetables**

  - Collard greens*
  - Dandelion greens
  - Mixed greens
  - Mustard greens
  - Red, yellow, and green peppers
  - Onions*
  - Mushrooms
  - Spinach
  - Carrots

  - Radishes
  - Kale*
  - Broccoli*
  - Swiss chard*
  - Brussels sprouts*
  - Asparagus*
  - Cabbage*
  - Cucumbers
  - Celery
  - Red beets (Beets may be steamed for 20-30 minutes or until soft. Patients may use the beet greens in salads after washing.)

  *May be steamed for four minutes

- **Salads with unlimited fresh vegetables**

  - Salad dressings are **not** permissible
  - Nuts, seeds, and beans (including green beans) are **not** permissible

Detoxification

- **Fruit – eat twice as many vegetables as compared to fruit (1 serving = 1 cup)**

    - Examples include but are not limited to:
        - Apples
        - Oranges
        - Bananas
        - Grapes
        - Berries
        - Melons
        - Tomatoes

        Avocadoes are not permissible

- **2 servings of brown or wild rice (not instant) per day (1 serving = 1 cup)**

- **Spring water (at least 8 glasses per day)**

REFRAIN FROM HAVING THE PATIENT CONSUME ANYTHING NOT LISTED
When followed as directed, this purification program has shown in clinical practice to offer great rewards in terms of desired outcomes and patient satisfaction. Any alteration of the instructions allows for variables that could decrease the benefits of the program; therefore, it is recommended that the instructions are followed completely and not modified.

Supplementation

SP Complete™ and Gastro-Fiber® are recommended throughout the entire program; SP Cleanse® is recommended for week one only; and SP Green Food™ is recommended for weeks two and three.

Week One
- 2-3 SP Complete shakes per day
  (refer to the last page of this section for the shake recipe)
- 7 SP Cleanse capsules 3 times daily without food/but with shakes or water
- 3 Gastro-Fiber capsules 3 times daily without food/but with shakes or water

Weeks Two & Three
- 2-3 SP Complete shakes per day
- 3 Gastro-Fiber capsules 3 times daily without food/but with shakes or water
- 5 SP Green Food capsules 2 times daily without food/but with shakes or water

PLEASE NOTE THAT SUPPLEMENTS SHOULD BE TAKEN WITH AN SP COMPLETE SHAKE OR WATER, BUT NOT WITH FOOD. THE SUPPLEMENTS MAY ALSO BE TAKEN RIGHT BEFORE BED.

Exercise
It is recommended that your patients walk at least four times per week for 30-45 minutes. Strenuous exercise should be put on hold during the three-week period.

SP Complete™ Supplement Shake Recipe

1 - 1½ cups of fruit
8 oz. of water (increase for desired consistency)
1 tablespoon flaxseed oil
2 rounded scoops (tablespoons) of SP Complete

Directions:
Thoroughly blend all ingredients together. Patients may make a large enough batch to last through the day, but make sure to keep it refrigerated, and remix it as needed before pouring.

Dysbiosis

Defined

Dysbiosis is the decrease in the number of favorable intestinal bacteria and subsequent increase in unfavorable organisms.

Signs and Symptoms

- Foul smelling bowel gas
- Bloating
- Abdominal pain
- Alternating diarrhea and constipation

Etiology and Contributing Factors

- Fungal overgrowth
- Impaired digestion
- Inadequate liver and gallbladder functioning
- Low-fiber diet
- Decreased immune function
- Altered stool pH
- Poor food choices (e.g. lack of essential fatty acids; fried foods, processed foods)
- Food additives (e.g. dyes, MSG, nitrates)
- Eating before going to bed
- Not chewing thoroughly
- Tap water (e.g. fluoride, chlorine)
- Antibiotics (prescribed or added to foods) or drug therapy
- High-protein diets
- High refined sugar intake
- Stress
- Hypothyroidism
- Intestinal parasites

Treatment Considerations

First address the cause of the gut flora dysbiosis. Once this has been addressed, reseed the bowel with a probiotic. The two most important types of flora to set the stage for a healthy intestinal environment are *Lactobacillus acidophilus* and *Bifidobacterium bifidum.*

Supplementation

Primary Support

The following two protocols both provide support for the dysbiotic bowel. Choose the one that best meets the needs of your particular case.

Protocol One

Zymex® (Capsules) (Standard Process): Specialized yeast culture that does not produce CO_2 and supports the formation of lactic acid from carbohydrates in the large intestine which results in lowering the pH of the stool. Overall effect is to promote a healthy balance of intestinal flora and create an environment not conducive to fungal overgrowth.

Dosage: Two capsules, three times per day with meals. Finish the entire bottle.

Dysbiosis

Note: For patients with lactose intolerance, please note that Zymex® does contain lactose; so use the alternate product Lactic Acid Yeast™ (Standard Process) instead of Zymex®. These are in a wafer form with the dosage being two to three wafers three times per day with meals. Lactic Acid Yeast™ can be used when or after a patient has been on antibiotic therapy. Patients should take two to three wafers three times per day with meals and continue this for one week post-antibiotic therapy along with two to three Lact-Enz® per day(between meals). (See below for information regarding the usage of Lact-Enz®.)

LactEnz® (Standard Process): A probiotic that is a source of *Lactobacillus acidophilus* and *Bifidobacterium bifidum* along with protease, amylase, lipase, and cellulase.

Dosage: Three capsules two to three times per day at least one hour before or two hours after a meal is suggested. Taking the capsules between meals ensures maximum delivery of the probiotic into the small and large intestine. Finish the entire bottle.

Protocol Two

For two consecutive days of the week:

Garlic 5000mg (MediHerb): Traditionally used as a broad-spectrum antimicrobial agent.

Dosage: One tablet, three to four times per day.

> AND

Vitanox (MediHerb): The tannins in this product are poorly absorbed in the gastrointestinal tract and are thus carried to the large bowel. Tannins have the capacity to bind proteins; therefore they can inhibit the growth of all microorganisms, but appear to be specifically selective for the pathogenic organisms.

Dosage: One tablet, two to three times per day.

For the other five days of the week:

Gastro-Fiber® (Standard Process): A source of apple pectin and psyllium to encourage healthy microflora.

Dosage: Three capsules, three times per day with meals.

> OR

Aloe Vera 4.5:1 (MediHerb): Aloe Vera selectively encourages the growth of healthy microflora.

Dosage: Twenty-five mL, three times a day.

Additional herbs to consider:

Golden Seal 500mg (MediHerb): Broad-spectrum antimicrobial herb.

Dosage: One tablet, two to three times per day.

Marshmallow Root 1:5 Glycetract (MediHerb): Used as a pre-biotic to encourage growth of healthy microflora.

Dosage: Three mL, once or twice per day.

Dysmenorrhea (Spasmodic, Congestive)

Defined

Dysmenorrhea is mild, moderate, or severe menstrual pain classified as either primary or secondary.

1. Primary dysmenorrhea has no structural pathology associated with its etiology. It is divided into two etiological classifications, spasmodic and/or congestive.

2. Secondary dysmenorrhea is the sequalae to some pathology; such as uterine fibroids or endometriosis.

This protocol will focus on primary dysmenorrhea, however, these guidelines will also be of value for patients with secondary dysmenorrhea, along with the specific recommendations for the related pathology. (For dysmenorrhea associated with endometriosis or fibroids, please refer to these specific protocols for additional support.)

Symptoms

There are two types of pain patterns associated with primary dysmenorrhea:

1. Spasmodic dysmenorrhea

- Lower abdominal pain, usually presents as cramp-like, but can also be a dull, constant ache that radiates to the lower back or legs.
- Pain can begin shortly before menses or with menses, peaking within approximately 24 hours and usually subsiding after two days.
- Headache, constipation, nausea, diarrhea, and increased urinary frequency are common.
- In more severe cases, vomiting may be present.

2. Congestive dysmenorrhea

- Pain is described as dull, heavy, and constant.
- Pain is normally located in the lower pelvic region; however, it often radiates to the lower back or upper thighs.
- Pain may start late in the luteal phase and/or continue through the beginning of menses.

Most women experience a combination of both spasmodic and congestive dysmenorrhea.

Etiology

- Pain due to spasmodic uterine contractions and ischemia is most often mediated by the prostaglandins released from the secretory endometrium. It is for this reason that primary dysmenorrhea is usually associated with ovulatory cycles.
- Inadequate estrogen production resulting in progesterone dominance.
- Inadequate hepatic clearance of female reproductive hormones.
- Stress (emotional and physical).
- Compromised circulation resulting in endometrial ischemia.

Treatment Considerations

When addressing the hormone imbalance of dysmenorrhea consider the following:

- Provide nutritional support for the uterus to normalize uterine muscle activity.
- Address uterine ischemia by enhancing blood flow.
- Balance the synthesis of anti-inflammatory and pro-inflammatory prostaglandins.
- Provide analgesic and antispasmodic remedies for pain.
- Provide liver support to ensure adequate metabolism and breakdown of hormones.

Dysmenorrhea (Spasmodic, Congestive)

- Address emotional distress with nervine tonics and make use of adaptogens when stress, anxiety, and/or depression are present.
- Address hormone imbalance.

Supplementation for Primary Dysmenorrhea

Primary Support

Utrophin PMG® (Standard Process): Specific uterine tissue support utilizing Protomorphogen™ extracts.

Dosage: One to two tablets, three times per day with meals.

Cramplex (MediHerb): A combination of herbal extracts which provides the following actions:

- Acts as a uterine tonic
- Reduces uterine pain
- Anti-spasmodic activity
- Relieves congestion in the uterus
- Reduces nausea and diarrhea
- Anti-inflammatory

Dosage: Two tablets, every three-four hours, four times per day.

Note: Start two to three days prior to menses. If the patient has begun her cycle and is experiencing cramping, she can start with the above dosage. The patient can discontinue Cramplex once the pain is gone.

Dong Quai (MediHerb): Uterine tonic which helps remove circulatory congestion of the reproductive organs by reducing platelet aggregation. This herb is particularly effective with congestive dysmenorrhea.

Dosage: One tablet, three times per day.

Warning: Contraindicated in bleeding disorders. If patient has a very heavy menstrual flow, use Dong Quai on non-bleeding days of the cycle only. If she has a scant menstrual flow, Dong Quai can be used throughout the cycle.

Wheat Germ Oil (Standard Process): Rich source of the whole vitamin E complex. Vitamin E is helpful in reducing blood stagnation and clotting. Vitamin E also reduces painful inflammations caused by leukotriene production from arachidonic acid and supports oxygen delivery to the uterine tissue which helps ease congestion.

Dosage: Two perles, three times per day with meals.

Ginkgo 2000mg (MediHerb): For relief of uterine congestion.

Dosage: One tablet, three times per day.

Secondary Support: As Indicated

If the patient is under significant stress, suffering from depression and/or anxiety, their hormone balance can be affected. Consider one or a combination of the following products.

- **Valerian Complex (MediHerb):** Helps ease the effects of stress and anxiety on the body. A natural calmative for both muscle and nervous tension.

  Dosage: One tablet, three to four times per day.

- **Nevaton® (MediHerb):** Nervine tonic for effects of depression and anxiety. This formula also provides adaptogenic support for the liver and adrenal glands.

  Dosage: One tablet, three to four times per day.

Dysmenorrhea (Spasmodic, Congestive)

- **Chaste Tree (MediHerb):** Helps increase luteinizing hormone levels and reduces prolactin levels. Overall effect is to ensure that ovulation takes place so that normal endogenous progesterone levels are maintained.

  ### When to use Chaste Tree:

  I. Dysmenorrhea without PMS: Chaste Tree is contra-indicated and can exacerbate symptoms. If the woman is experiencing dysmenorrhea without other cyclical premenstrual complaints, then she is potentially progesterone dominant. For this situation, utilization of estrogen modulating herbs is appropriate.

  II. Dysmenorrhea with PMS: If other premenstrual symptoms occur along with the dysmenorrhea, then **Chaste Tree is indicated.**

  Dosage: Two tablets, once per day in the morning.

  ### Herb-Drug Interaction: Pertaining to Chaste Tree and HRT

  I. Chaste Tree is best not taken in conjunction with progesterone drugs, hormone replacement therapy or the contraceptive pill. For these situations, substitute either Standard Process **Ovex**® (one to two tablets three times per day with meals throughout cycle) or MediHerb's **White Peony** 1:2 (Four mL per day throughout cycle).

  II. Chaste Tree, Ovex®, and White Peony can be used long term.

- **LivCo® (MediHerb):** Supports liver detoxification by enhancing the cytochrome P450 phase I and phase II pathways. The desired effect is to enhance hepatic clearance of hormones.

  Dosage: One tablet, three times per day.

- **White Peony 1:2 (MediHerb):** Restores normal hormonal balance through its support of folliculogenesis.

  Dosage: Four mL per day throughout the cycle. Can be used long term.

Calcium Lactate (Standard Process): Calcium is necessary for smooth and skeletal muscle contraction and relaxation. Add calcium to any of the above products when cramping is not totally resolved with specific protocols.

Dosage: For severe cases, recommend two tablets four times per day. Best taken on an empty stomach.

Emphysema

Defined

A lung condition typically characterized by an above normal increase in the size of air spaces, distal to the terminal bronchiole (those parts containing alveoli), with destructive changes in their walls and reduction in their number. Obstruction results from changes within the tissue rather than mucus production, which occurs in asthma and bronchitis. The distinguishing characteristic of emphysema is the airflow limitation that results by lack of elastic recoil in the lungs. There are three types of emphysema: centrilobular, panlobular, and distal acinar.

Centrilobular emphysema: The distinctive feature of this type of emphysema is the pattern of involvement of the lobules: the proximal or central parts of the acini, formed by the respiratory bronchioles, are affected, while the distal alveoli are spared. The result is that both normal and emphysematous airspaces exist with the same acinus and lobule. The lesions tend to be more severe and common in the upper lobes. In severe centrilobular emphysema the distal acinus also is involved, and as a result, the differentiation from panlobular emphysema becomes difficult.

Panlobular emphysema: In this type of emphysema the acini are enlarged (uniformly) from the level of the respiratory bronchiole to the terminal blind alveoli. Panacinar emphysema tends to occur in the lower lung zones and is the type of emphysema that occurs in alpha-1-trypsin deficiency.

Distal Acinar: In this form of emphysema the proximal portion of the acinus is normal but the distal part is mainly involved. The emphysema is more prevalent adjacent to the pleura, along the lobular connective tissue septa, and at the margins of the lobules. It occurs next to areas of fibrosis, atelectasis, or scarring and is usually more severe in the upper half of the lungs.

Symptoms & Signs

- Dyspnea on exertion
- Barrel chest
- Tachypenea
- Prolonged expiration and grunting
- Decreased chest expansion
- Clubbed fingers and toes
- Hyperresonance
- Decreased breath sounds
- Crackles and wheezing on inspiration
- Symptoms of chronic bronchitis may often, but not necessarily, coexist

Etiology

- Aging - senile emphysema is the result of degenerative changes that cause stretching without destruction of the smooth muscle. The connective tissue is usually not affected.
- Smoking of marijuana
- Alpha-1-antitrypsin deficiency
- Cigarette smoking
- Inhalation of chemical pollutants
- Free radicals - excessive production of free radicals can damage the alveoli of the lungs and result in inhibiting antitrypsin production.
- Particulate exposure – e.g. mining dust, micro-fibers in asbestos (asbestosis), fiberglass insulation, diesel exhaust, silica, metal grinders

Emphysema

Treatment Considerations

- Provide nutritional factors needed to support healing and maintenance of the affected tissues
- Remove offending agents
- Employ bronchial dilating herbs
- Use of anti-catarrhal and mucolytic remedies to reduce mucus production when necessary
- Antitussives and expectorants may be necessary if the case dictates

Supplementation

Note: Progress with whole food and herbal treatments in emphysema depends on the extent of alveoli damage. Emphysema is extremely difficult to reverse.

Primary Support

Emphaplex® (Standard Process): A combination formula designed to support the pulmonary system. Specific factors in this product include mucolytic factors, lung Protomorphogen™ extract, adrenal support, essential amino acids, protein metabolizing factors, and Catalyn®.

Dosage: Three capsules, three times per day with meals.

ResCo or ResCo Phytosynergist™ (MediHerb): Provides the following actions: expectorant, demulcent, antispasmodic, and diaphoretic activity.

Dosage: Resco – Four to six tablets per day. Duration of use is six weeks on and two weeks off, etc.
    Or
    ResCo Phytosynergist™ – Five mL three times per day. Duration of use is six weeks on and two weeks off, etc.

OPC Synergy (Standard Process): Indicated for emphysema due to its ability to support airway architecture. The Oligoproanthocyanadins (OPCs) protect against free radical damage and support alveoli structure.

Dosage: One capsule, three times per day with meals.

Cataplex® E2 (Standard Process): This product is useful in alleviating tissue oxygen starvation caused by poor lung capacity. The E2 fraction of the vitamin E complex is a phospholipid. Cataplex® E2 may help oxygen delivery by enhancing the permeability of the cell membrane.

Dosage: One to two tablets, three times daily with meals.

Secondary Support: As Indicated

For patients with pulmonary edema, see the section titled *Heart Failure* for additional information and protocols.

For patients with low blood oxygen carrying capacity, see the section titled *Anemia* for additional information and protocols.

Endometriosis

Defined

A nonmalignant disorder in which functioning endometrial tissue is found outside the uterine cavity.

Endometriosis is usually restricted to the peritoneal or serosal surfaces of the abdominal organs, most commonly the posterior broad ligament, ovaries, uterosacral ligaments, and posterior cul-de-sac. Less common sites include the bladder, vagina, pleura, pericardium, surgical scars, ureters, and serosal surfaces of the small and large intestine. When endometrial tissue is found in the ovaries, this can lead to the formation of cysts after the tissue becomes encapsulated. As with normal endometrium, any tissue located outside the uterus remains under the influence of hormones, causing it to bleed during menses and eventually leading to the formation of scar tissue and adhesions.

Signs and Symptoms

- Classic symptoms include dysmennorhea, infertility, and abnormal uterine bleeding
- Pain – typically begins 5-7 days before menses, peaks, and lasts for 2 to 3 days (the severity does not reflect the extent of the disease)
- Depending on the site of the ectopic tissue:
    - ovaries and oviducts: profuse menses, infertility
    - cul de sac or ovaries: deep-thrust dyspareunia
    - bladder: dysuria, suprapubic pain, hematuria
    - large bowel, appendix: pain on defecation, abdominal cramps, constipation; bloody stools
    - cervix, perineum, vagina: bleeding from endometrial deposits, painful intercourse

Etiology

Suggested causes (one or more may be applicable in different women):

- Depressed immune system and genetic predisposition
- Retrograde menstruation with implantation of endometrial tissue at ectopic sites
- Hematogenous or lymphatic spread to extraperitoneal sites

Note: Ectopic endometrial tissue can become implanted almost anywhere in the pelvic peritoneum. It can even invade remote sites such as the lungs.

Treatment Considerations

- Modulate estrogen levels
- Administer progesterogenic remedies
- Provide nutritional support for the endometrial tissue
- Use spasmolytic agents
- Use anti-hemorrhagic agents
- Reduce inflammation

Endometriosis

Supplementation

Primary Support

Utrophin PMG® (Standard Process): Specific support for the uterus utilizing *Protomorphogen*™ extracts.

Dosage: One tablet, three times per day with meals.

Chaste Tree (MediHerb): Supports proper ovulation resulting in balancing the relative ratio of progesterone to estrogen during the luteal phase of the menstrual cycle.

Dosage: Four to six tablets per day (divide the dosage between morning and evening).

Wheat Germ Oil (Standard Process): A rich source of the whole vitamin E complex. This source of the vitamin E complex traditionally has been helpful in reducing blood stagnation and clotting. Vitamin E also reduces painful inflammation caused by leukotrine production from arachidonic acid and helps increase oxygen delivery to the uterine tissue to help ease congestion.

Dosage: Two perles, three times per day with meals.

Evening Primrose Oil (MediHerb): Anti-inflammatory due to its high content of Gamma-linolenic Acid (GLA). Evening Primrose Oil supports the body's production of Dihomogamma-linolenic Acid (DGLA). This occurs as a result of the GLA in the Evening Primrose Oil being converted to Dihommogamma-linoleinc Acid (DGLA) from which our body makes the series 1 prostaglandins.

Dosage: One capsule, three times per day.

This protocol can be used long term and may need to be continued until the patient is in full menopause. Once the patient reaches menopause, the influence of estrogen on endometrial tissue is significantly reduced. Gradually reduce the dose of remedies post menopause over a three-month period to allow the body to readapt.

Secondary Support: As Indicated

Symplex® F (Standard Process): Pituitary, thyroid, adrenal and ovary support utilizing *Protomorphogen*™ extracts. Use this product when more broad-based endocrine support is needed. Use in conjunction with Utrophin PMG®.

Dosage: One to two tablets, three times per day with meals.

Capsella Complex Phytosynergist™ (MediHerb): Consider this formula for heavy painful periods. Allow 2-3 cycles to see maximum benefits.

Dosage: Five mL, three times per day. Start taking 2-3 days prior to menses and discontinue at the cessation of menses. This regimen can be used long term and should be continued every month.

For additional pain and anti-inflammatory support consider one of the following:

Cramplex (MediHerb): Provides the following actions:

- Acts as a uterine tonic
- Reduces uterine pain
- Provides anti-spasmodic activity
- Relieves congestion in the uterus
- Acts as an anti-inflammatory

Dosage: Two tablets every three to four hours, four times per day.

It is best to start 2-3 days prior to menses and discontinue after the first 24 days of menses. If the patient has already begun her cycle and is experiencing discomfort, have her begin taking Cramplex immediately. Cramplex can be discontinued once the pain has subsided for twenty-four hours.

Endometriosis

Boswellia Complex (MediHerb): The synergistic properties of the herbs in this formula support the body's removal of inflammatory acidic metabolic waste products and also provide anti-inflammatory and depurative actions.

Dose: One to two tablets, three times daily.

Clinical Note: Hepatic clearance of endogenous estrogen as well as xenoestrogens (foreign compounds which mimic estrogen) is important in the nutritional treatment of endometriosis. Consider prescribing three to four tablets per day of LivCo (MediHerb). This product up regulates liver detoxification mechanisms for optimum hepatic clearance of estrogens.

Note: If using LivCo long term, make sure that the patient has a diet rich in liver-supporting foods to support optimal hepatic functioning. If their diet is insufficient in this respect, then refer to the section titled *General Liver Support*.

Enteric Infection

Defined

An enteric infection is an infection of the intestinal tract which may be caused by worms, viruses, amoeba, bacteria, or other parasites.

Signs and Symptoms

- Constipation
- Diarrhea
- Fever
- Fatigue
- Flatulence
- Foul smelling stools
- Food intolerance
- Hives
- Headaches
- Abdominal pain and cramps
- Abdominal bloating
- Indigestion
- Irregular bowel movements
- Increased intestinal permeability
- Loss of appetite
- Low back pain
- Weight loss
- Malabsorption
- Irritable bowel syndrome

Etiology

Each one of the microbial inhabitants of the gastrointestinal tract is a potential pathogenic parasite. Most clinicians consider protozoa and helminthes (roundworms, flatworms, flukes) as the primary agents.

Experts approximate that there are over 300 different varieties of parasites. The CDC estimates the number, however, to be in the thousands. They are divided into a few main categories.

1. **Roundworms (nematodes):** Intestinal roundworms can come from the eggs or larvae in fecal contaminated soil, contaminated vegetables, or cysts that reside in infected pork. Some common conditions that arise from intestinal roundworm infections are Ascariasis, Hookworm infection, Strongyloidiasis, Trichuriasis, and Enterobiasis.

2. **Protozoa:** These single-celled microscopic organisms are among the most common causes of disease and death in developing countries. In industrialized countries, protozoa are prevalent but less lethal (e.g. *Entamoeba histolytica, Giardia lamblia,* Trichomonas, and Toxoplasma). The most common intestinal protozoa are Entamoeba histolytica and Giardia lamblia. Each of these has two forms: (1) motile trophozites that can attach to the intestinal epithelial wall and may penetrate and (2) immobile cysts, which are infectious when eaten because they have a covering (chitin) that is resistant to stomach acids. Protozoan infections are from oral ingestion of a protozoan cyst which resides in the feces. *Entamoeba histolytica* and *Giardia lamblia* can be obtained via water supplies, such as contaminated swimming and recreational areas, diaper changing, poor food preparation, and through contact with infected animals. Trichomonas is the simplest protozoan parasite and is sexually transmitted and colonizes the male urethra and vagina. Additional examples of intestinal protozoan infectious agents are Entamoeba coli, Balantidium coli, Dientamoeba fragilis, and Toxoplasma gondi.

Note: *Trichomonas vaginalis* is a protozoan infection whose mode of transmission is through vaginal and prostatic secretions with the site of infection in the original host being the vagina and prostate.

3. **Tapeworm:** Source is usually larvae, cysts, or eggs from uncooked beef, fish, or pork. Ingestion is usually through the mouth.

Note: Tapeworms cannot be addressed with natural products.

4. **Flukes:** Intestinal infection is the result of *Fasciolopsis buski* from contaminated water, nuts, and/or vegetables.

Enteric Infection

The rise in international travel coupled with a compromised internal terrain due to the use of antibiotics (prescription and in the food supply), immunosuppressive drugs, inadequate digestive enzymes, utilization of antacid medications, and the ingestion of foods laden with chemicals and sugar, leaves the host susceptible to an enteric infection.

Treatment Considerations

- Utilization of anthelmintics and proteolytic enzymes
- Support immune function with nutrition and immune enhancing herbs
- Establish optimum gastric and stool pH
- Promote elimination of larvae or damaged pathogenic organisms and eggs via the bowel

Supplementation

Primary Support

Use all the products in the primary protocol as instructed for twelve weeks for best results. Consider that a dysbiotic bowel may exist after addressing an enteric infection; in those cases, refer to the section titled *Dysbiosis* for further information.

Wormwood Complex (MediHerb): Each tablet of Wormwood Complex contains:

- Wormwood leaf (100 mg)
- Black Walnut hulls (100 mg)
- Stemona root (1000 mg)
- Clove Bud essential oil (20 mg)

These ingredients are well known for their anthelmintic activity. This herbal blend is a very potent remedy for the control of intestinal parasites by reducing motility, bursting the cell walls of larvae, and inhibiting reproduction. Additionally, the formula will provide a soothing carminative effect to the G.I. tract and have a beneficial effect on the production of digestive enzymes.

Dosage: Two to three tablets, twice daily <u>before meals</u> for first the 10 days and then repeat after a 10-day break.

OPC Synergy™ (Standard Process) or Vitanox (MediHerb): The tannin-containing herbs in OPC Synergy™ and Vitanox (green tea and grape seed extract) act as synergists to cause the bursting of worm larvae when combined with Clove oil.

Dosage: OPC Synergy™ - One to two capsules taken along with Wormwood Complex, but separate from Zymex® II by at least two hours.
Or
Vitanox - One to two tablets taken along with Wormwood Complex, but separate from Zymex® II by at least two hours.

Zymex® II (Standard Process): Provides papain, bromelain, fig powder, and almond powder. These are natural proteolytic enzymes that when given on an empty stomach, will support the breakdown of pathogenic microflora that may exist in the gastrointestinal tract. In addition to its potent array of proteolytic enzymes from plants, Zymex II contains ficin. Sources of ficin have been used traditionally in the Amazon as an anthelmintic.

Dosage: Two to three capsules, three times per day <u>between meals</u>.

Garlic 5000mg (Mediherb): Anthelmintic, antifungal, and mucolytic.

Dosage: One tablet, two to three times per day with meals.

Enteric Infection

Spanish Black Radish *(Organically Grown)* **(Standard Process):** Due to its high sulfur content, Spanish Black Radish creates an intestinal environment that does not support parasitic growth.

Dosage: Two tablets, three times per day with meals.

Note: After 30 days on the above program, then add introduce Lact-Enz®.

LactEnz® (Standard Process): Probiotic used to maintain healthy intestinal flora. Lact-Enz® provides lactobacilli and Bifidobacterium and is prepared in such a way that it does not require refrigeration to maintain its bioactivity. Lact-Enz is also a source proteolytic plant and pancreatic enzymes.

Dosage: Three capsules two times per day at least one hour before or two hours after a meal. Taking the capsules between meals ensures maximum delivery of the probiotic into the intestines.

General Recommendations

1. Reduce protein quantity to approximately 4-5 oz. per meal. The aim is to have the proteolytic enzymes digesting pathogens not food. This will increase effectiveness of the program.
2. Drink at least eight glasses of filtered spring water per day – NOT tap water!
3. Avoid refined sugar products and high glycemic foods, such as juices.
4. Bowel movements should be a minimum of once daily.

Secondary Support: As Indicated

Zypan® (Standard Process): It is always important to be careful about what you eat. Should you eat food that is either improperly handled and/or cooked, then you stand the risk of developing an enteric infection. In order to promote the gastric acid barrier, adequate proteolytic enzymes along with the proper gastric pH is vital in order to help prevent the infiltration of parasitic organisms into the gastrointestinal tract. Zypan® provides the following factors, pepsin, betaine hydrochloride, ammonium chloride, and pancreatic enzymes which provide the proteolytic enzymes and acidity needed to facilitate a healthy functioning upper gastrointestinal tract.

Dosage: Two tablets <u>with meals</u>

Note: Multizyme® (Standard Process) Provides enzymatic support for protein, fat, and starch digestion. This is a good alternative to Zypan® when additional acidity is contraindicated in the gastric region. Both Multizyme® and Zypan® can be used simultaneously if needed.

Dosage: Two capsules three times per day with meals.

Immuplex® (Standard Process): Provides the vitamin A, C, and E complexes, folic acid, cyanocobalamin, trace minerals, and liver, thymus, spleen, and bone Protomorphogen™ extracts along with other synergistic factors for optimal immune system support. This is not a product to be used for an acute case but rather for those with depleted immune systems that require the nutritional factors to optimize the immune response.

Dosage: Two capsules three times per day with meals.

Andrographis Complex (MediHerb): Immune enhancing through the combined action of *Echinacea angustifolia*, *Andrographis paniculata*, and Holy Basil.

Dosage: One tablet three times per day.

Uterine Fibroids

Defined

Benign muscular tumor(s), located in the uterus, are composed of smooth muscle and fibrous tissue. The most common sites are submucosal, subserosal, and intramural. Fibroids can, however, occur in the uterine tubes or broad ligaments (intraligamentous).

Signs and Symptoms

- Often assymptomatic
- Menorrhagia (most common symptom)
- Metrorrhagia
- Severe pain or pressure (from growth, hemorrhage, degeneration, or twisting of a pedunculated fibroid)
- Urinary or bowel complaints (e.g., constipation, urinary urgency or frequency)
- Infertility
- Recurrent abortions
- Anemia from heavy bleeding

Etiology

The cause of fibroid growth is unknown. High estrogen levels appear to stimulate their growth. Since uterine fibroid growth is affected by estrogen, they will be aggravated by excess estrogen. Relative estrogen excess can be the result of:

- Xenobiotic exposure through a diet of non-organic, non-free range foods
- Anovulatory cycles
- Hormone replacement therapy
- Relative progesterone deficiency
- Nutritional deficiencies
- Low-fiber diet
- Reduced hepatic clearance of estrogen

Treatment Considerations

- Control fibroid growth and alleviate symptoms associated by the fibroids. Chaste tree is the herb of choice and can be given in high doses to reduce estrogen production if the fibroids are severe.
- Use of anti-hemorrhagic agents to control the heavy irregular bleeding
- The use of estrogen modulating remedies in older women who tend to ovulate less frequently may be indicated. Estrogen modulating herbs such as wild yam and false unicorn which encourage ovulation should only be used in conjunction with chaste tree for fibroids and not in high doses.
- Since estrogen has an effect on fibroid tissue, hepatic functioning should be optimal in order to breakdown and remove estrogen and xenobiotics through the appropriate mechanisms. Refer to the sections titled **General Liver Support** or **Detoxification** for further reading.
- Uterine support with the appropriate *Protomorphogen*™ extracts

Supplementation

Primary Support

Utrophin PMG® (Standard Process): Specific support for the uterus utilizing *Protomorphogen*™ extracts.

Dosage: One to two tablets, three times per day with meals.

Chaste Tree (MediHerb): Supports proper ovulation resulting in balancing the relative ratio of estrogen to progesterone during the luteal phase of the menstrual cycle.

Dosage: Two to three tablets in the morning and two to three tablets in the evening.

Wheat Germ Oil (Standard Process): Rich source of the vitamin E complex. This source of the vitamin E complex is helpful in reducing blood stagnation and clotting. Vitamin E also reduces painful inflammation caused by leukotrine production from arachidonic acid and helps increase oxygen delivery to the uterine tissue to help ease congestion.

Dosage: Two perles, three times per day with meals.

Note: *Since the tumors are estrogen dependent, treatment may need to be continued until the women is in full menopause.*

Echinacea Premium (MediHerb): Traditionally used to suppress progress of benign growths.

Dosage: One tablet, three times per day.

Capsella Complex Phytosynergist™ (MediHerb): Consider this formula for heavy painful periods. Allow 2-3 cycles to see maximum benefits.

Dosage: Five to ten mL, three times per day. Start taking 2-3 days prior to menses and discontinue when menses ceases. This regimen is continued every month. This formula can be used long term.

Secondary Support: As Indicated

Symplex® F (Standard Process): Pituitary, thyroid, adrenal and ovarian support utilizing *Protomorphogen*™ extracts. Use in conjunction with Utrophin PMG® if more broad based endocrine support is needed.

Dosage: One tablet, three times daily.

Ginkgo 2000 mg (MediHerb): For relief of uterine congestion.

Dosage: One tablet, three times per day.

Note: *If anemia is an issue with a particular case, consider the following in addition to the above primary support remedies.*

Ferrofood® *or* Fe-Max Iron Tonic Phytosynergist™

- **Ferrofood® (Standard Process):** Supplies iron in an assimilable form (ferrous lactate) along with other synergistic cofactors that provide the nutrients needed to support optimal red blood cell production.

  Dosage: One to two capsules, three times per day with meals.

- **Fe-Max Iron Tonic Phytosynergist™ (MediHerb):** Blend of herbs, vitamins, and minerals to promote and support normal blood cell production and improve assimilation of iron from foods. The bitters in this formula improve gastric acid production. This product should also be considered for the vegetarian. Also for the vegetarian, consider using 5-10 mL/day of MediHerb's Ashwaganda 1:2 (Ashwaganda root 1:2 extract from *Withania somnifera* root 2.5g) as an alternative to Ferrofood® along with Fe-Max Iron TonicPhytosynergist™. Ashwaganda helps promote normal RBC production.

  Dosage: Five mL, three times per day.

Utilize two bottles of Fe-Max Iron Tonic Phytosynergist™ at the above dosage, then monitor blood iron levels. If unable to monitor blood levels, provide one bottle every three to four months at the above dosage. For women with monthly heavy menstrual flow, the recommended dosage would be 5 mL, once per day long term. Again, periodic monitoring of blood iron levels is advised.

Chlorophyll Complex™ (Standard Process): Used traditionally as a blood builder due to the similarity of the porphyrin ring of chlorophyll to the heme molecule.

Dosage: Two perles, three times per day to be used along with Ferrofood® or Fe-Max Iron Tonic Phytosynergist™.

Food Allergies

Defined

A food allergy is an allergic response to a specific protein in food(s) in which the body generates an antibody-antigen complex.

Note: Food allergies are often confused with a food intolerance which is when the body does not have the capacity to digest or breakdown certain foods correctly.

Signs and Symptoms

Patients can have a broad range of different reactions when faced with an allergen. Symptoms can also range from mild to life threatening and may occur immediately or remain masked for days. Some common reactions include:

- Eczema
- Migraine headaches
- Colitis
- Arthritis (rheumatic pain)
- Asthma
- Enuresis (night time bed wetting)
- Urticaria (hives often attended by itching)

Etiology

Protein denaturation as defined in the 28th edition of *Dorlands Illustrated Medical Dictionary* is any disruption of the configuration of a protein, as by heat, change in pH, or other physical means or chemical means, resulting in alteration of the physical properties and loss of biological activity of the protein. If this denaturation does not occur due to adequate digestive processes, then an allergic reaction to protein is possible.

It is important to remember that a foreign protein, once hydrolyzed to small peptides and amino acids, is no longer considered capable of provoking an immune response.

Additional predisposing factors:

- Genetic predisposition
- Genetic manipulation of food supply
- Excess gastrointestinal permeability
- Too little dietary diversity
- Poor digestion
- Poor liver function
- Food additives

Treatment Considerations

A nutritional approach to food allergies usually involves the following considerations:

- Detoxification
- Supporting digestive function
- Healing of the gastrointestinal tract (if indicated)
- Removal of offending foods

Food Allergies

Supplementation

Primary Support: Detoxification

Refer to the section titled *Detoxification*.

Primary Support: Digestive Support

Zypan® (Standard Process): Provides betaine hydrochloride, pepsin, and ammonium chloride along with pancreatic enzymes to support optimal protein, fat, and carbohydrate digestion. Consider this the primary Standard Process proteolytic product with some broad-based small intestinal digestive support added.

Dosage: One to two tablets per meal. Can be used long term.

Multizyme® (Standard Process): Provides enzymatic support for protein, fat, and starch digestion. This is a good alternative to Zypan® when additional acidity is contraindicated in the gastric region. *Both Multizyme® and Zypan® can be used simultaneously if so desired.*

Dosage: Two capsules, three times per day with meals. Can be used long term.

A-F Betafood® (Standard Process): Provides nutrients to support bile production and flow.

Dosage: Two to five tablets, three times per day with meals. Can be used long term.

Secondary Support

Antronex® (Standard Process): Liver extract that facilitates portal vein dilation and enhances hepatic clearance of histamine.

Dosage: Two tablets, three times per day with meals or two per hour for an acute case.

Phosfood® Liquid (Standard Process): Phosphorous is an acid ash mineral that supports the sympathetic nervous system. This is the branch of the autonomic nervous system that supports the immune organs that respond in an allergic response.

Dosage: Two droppers full, two to three times per day in a glass of water.

Clinical Notes

Doctors should advise patients to:
- Widen scope of ingested nutrients to include a variety of organic vegetables, fruits, and free range animal products.

The following is a simple test that can be used to assess ones response to particular foods:

Coca's Pulse Test for Food Allergies
1. Take the pulse before one consumes the food that you wish to test.
2. Have the patient maintain a relaxed position in a place where they don't feel stressed.
3. Wait at least twenty minutes and then take the pulse again. If the heart rate is ten beats higher (or more), an allergy may be the cause.

Gallstones (Cholelithiasis)

Defined

Accumulation of solid crystals (predominately cholesterol) in the bile ducts (biliary tree) or gallbladder. Choledocholithiasis is the presence of stones in the bile ducts and Cholelithiasis is the presence of the stones in the gallbladder.

Approximately 80% of stones are cholesterol stones, containing crystalline cholesterol monohydrate. The remainder are composed predominately of bilirubin calcium salts and are referred to as pigmented stones.

Signs and Symptoms

- The majority of patients who have gallstones are asymptomatic. Typically, the stone should pass from the gallbladder into the cystic and common bile duct, and if tiny enough, it will continue on into the small intestine.

- Nausea and vomiting can occur if the stone obstructs the cystic or bile duct. Obstruction by a stone can allow bacteria to flourish and quickly result in an infection within the ducts, which could cause abscesses in the liver. Signs of an infection may be chills, fever, and jaundice.

  Note: If an infection is present, it could result in septicemia. This is a serious condition, therefore, the appropriate referral should be considered.

- Transient cystic duct obstruction will result in colicky pain.

- A stone could persistently obstruct the outlet of the gallbladder or the cystic duct. This results in constant pain (biliary colic) in the upper abdomen on the right side under the ribs. This type of pain usually comes on gradually lasting from a half hour to twelve hours before resolving. A continued obstruction can cause the gallbladder to become inflamed (cholecystitis). With this, the pain is steady and may refer to the right shoulder blade. There could be an associated fever as well.

- Stones that obstruct the pancreatic duct can result in inflammation of the pancreas and pain.

- Belching, fullness, and bloating are associated with cholelithiasis.

- Postprandial fatty food intolerance.

- Gallbladder involvement can result in referred pain to the upper thoracic spine along with pain localized under the right shoulder blade and towards the midline.

Etiology

Cholesterol Stones

Bile is the main pathway that enables the body to rid itself of cholesterol either in a free form or as bile salts. Cholesterol is insoluble in water; however, it is rendered water-soluble by aggregation with lecithin and bile salts, which are co-secreted into the bile. When the concentration of cholesterol exceeds the capacity of bile to solubilize it, then cholesterol can nucleate into solid cholesterol monohydrate crystals (stones).

Three conditions must therefore be met for cholesterol gallstone formation:

1. Supersaturation of bile with cholesterol. Supersaturation can result from increased output of cholesterol or decreased output of the bile acids, lecithin, and water, resulting in precipitating out of cholesterol. It is important to remember that the composition of the organic material of bile is as follows: approximately 4% cholesterol, 50% bile acids, and 40% phosphatidylcholine.

Gallstones (Cholelithiasis)

2. Conditions must be present for nucleation (a starting point for stone formation).
3. Reduced motility of the gallbladder may be an etiological factor. Cholesterol needs to remain in the gallbladder long enough to precipitate into stones.

Risk Factors for Cholesterol Stones

- Females are thought to be predisposed to gallstones as a result of reduced bile acid production or increased cholesterol production due to estrogens.
- Pregnancy, the use of oral contraceptives or other factors that elevate estrogen levels.
- Obesity: Overweight people have increased output of cholesterol from the liver thus increasing the risk of forming a gallstone(s).
- Fast weight reduction: Rapid or sudden weight loss causes an increase in the concentration of cholesterol in the bile. Couple this with the concomitant reduction in bile acid secretion and the stage is set for gallstone formation.
- Gallbladder stasis: Gallbladder stasis is a major contributor in permitting the formation and enlargement of stones. As the bile is stored in the gallbladder, it becomes more concentrated. This may allow increased cholesterol saturation.
- Hyperlipidemia syndromes.
- Advancing age.
- Disorders of bile acid metabolism.
- Gastrointestinal tract malfunction: Bile acids are normally reabsorbed in the ileum. Reduced resorption of bile acids due to diseases (Crohn's, etc.) increases the risk for gallstone formation.
- Low-fiber diet: Fiber is needed to bind cholesterol for excretion in the feces.

Note: Greater than 80% of gallstones are silent and may be so for many decades.

Pigmented Stones

The presence of unconjugated bilirubin seems to increase the likelihood of pigmented stone formation. The precipitation occurs primarily as insoluble calcium bilirubinate salts.

Risk Factors Associated with Pigmented Stones

- Chronic hemolytic conditions
- Biliary infection
- Gastrointestinal disorders (e.g. Crohn's disease)

Treatment Considerations

Obviously, the best scenario is to avoid the formation of gallstones in the first place. Most people with gallstones are asymptomatic. However, once formed, treatment is aimed at increasing the solubility of cholesterol in the bile as well as supporting bile production and flow. Keep in mind that if the symptoms worsen or persist, medical evaluation should be considered.

Treatment should only be rendered utilizing agents that support bile production and flow if the patient has a non-calcified gallstone, patent cystic duct, and is not in need of surgery or lithotripsy.

Supplementation

Primary Support

A-F Betafood® (Standard Process): Provides the nutrients that are needed to ensure healthy hepatic production and flow of bile.

Dosage: Two to three tablets three times per day with meals. Increasing the dosage to five tablets three times per day may be required in certain cases.

Gallstones (Cholelithiasis)

Choline (Standard Process): Acts as a physiological detergent through its role in phosphatidylcholine formation.

Dosage: Two tablets three times per day with meals.

Disodium Phosphate (Standard Process): Gently stimulates bile production and flow.

Dosage: Three capsules two times per day with a glass of warm water.

Gastro-Fiber® (Standard Process): Source of soluble and insoluble dietary fiber.

Dosage: Three capsules three times per day with meals.

Note: This protocol is to be used for one month. After one month, long-term liver support (see below) to support healthy bile production and flow should be considered.

Secondary Support: As Indicated

A-F Betafood® or Betafood® (both Standard Process): A-F Betafood® supports bile production and flow through the use of various food factors such as beet root and beet leaves. Betafood® contains more beet root and beet leaf and is thus higher in betaine - the bile thinning factor that gives beets their red color.

Dosage: A-F Betafood® – Two tablets three times per day with meals.
Or
Betafood® – One to two tablets three times per day with meals.

Livaplex® (Standard Process): This formula is a combination of six individual Standard Process products which support the following actions: bile production and flow, bowel detoxification, liver decongestion due to lipotrophic factors, hepatic Protomorphogen™ extract support, and enhanced blood flow through the portal vein.

Dosage: Two to three capsules three times per day with food.

General Endocrine Support

As you will see from the following, the importance of addressing the endocrine system is not a new concept. In fact, providing the appropriate support for those difficult cases might be all that's needed in order to obtain true resolution of a particular problem. In other words, it may provide the catalyst required to promote the healing response.

"The endocrines are functionally basic to all principles of physiology; in fact, endocrinology is physiology, and no physician or surgeon can qualify adequately in any phase of medical science who is failing in knowledge of this subject. We must all be endocrinologists to practice successfully the art of healing, which is our paramount function." ("The Interrelation of the Endocrines and the Vegetative Nervous System," William V. Garretson, *New York Medical Journal,* March 15, 1922)

"Empirical evidence reveals to us that the causes of many local manifestations may be shown to lie in endocrine disorders, which cannot be diagnosed or treated by attention to any one part of the body. To not consider endocrine support, when the response to therapeutic measures is slow or minimal, is to ignore an important aspect of nutritional therapeutics. If the diagnosis of ulcer is proven, causation of the ulcer is still wholly obscure. Almost any neurologist can offer case reports in which ulcer or perforation of an ulcer seems to have been precipitated by an emotional state such as anxiety or fear. Focal infection has been ascribed as the cause of nearly every type of pathological condition. It has been demonstrated that the frequency of peptic and duodenal ulcer is very high in cats and dogs following total extirpation of the suprarenal glands. Certain abnormalities of the intestinal mucosa are perhaps occasioned by failure of the suprarenals Resection of the ulcer or other local measures may be, therefore, merely treatment of a symptom, when a more general endocrinopathy should be studied." ("The Relation of the General Practitioner to the Specialist" *West Virginia Medical Journal,* Nov., 1930, xxvi, p. 645)

Supplementation

This section differs from the rest of the manual. You will not need to recommend all the products under primary support as is the case with the rest of the manual; choose only the product(s) that best support each individual case.

Note: Since you are not feeding with Protomorphogen™ extracts, one should always recommend the appropriate food based supplement along with the prescribed Protomorphogen™ extract.

Primary Support: Hypothalamus

Hypothalamus PMG® (Standard Process): Hypothalamus Protomorphogen™ extract support.

Dosage: One to two tablets, three times per day with meals.

Hypothalmex® (Standard Process): Cytosol™ extract support for the hypothalamus.

Dosage: One to two tablets, three times per day with meals.

Primary Support: Pituitary, Thyroid, Adrenal, and Gonad

Symplex® F (Standard Process): Female Protomorphogen™ extract support for the pituitary, thyroid, adrenal glands, and ovaries.

Dosage: One to two tablets, three times per day with meals.

Symplex® M (Standard Process): Male Protomorphogen™ extract support for the pituitary, thyroid, adrenal glands, and testicles.

Dosage: One to two tablets, three times per day with meals.

Primary Support: Pituitary

Pituitrophin PMG® (Standard Process): Pituitary Protomorphogen™ extract support

Dosage: One to two tablets, three times per day with meals.

Neuroplex® (Standard Process): Source of pituitary Protomorphogen™ extract, desiccated spleen, hypothalamus, and anterior pituitary. Rich source of *Tillandsia usneoides,* thiamine, niacin, riboflavin, iron, zinc, and copper as well as cofactors to help support maximize oxygen delivery via the blood to the brain.

Dosage: One to three capsules, three times per day.

Neurotrophin PMG® (Standard Process): Protomorphogen™ extract support for brain and nerve tissue.

Dosage: One to two tablets, three times per day with meals.

Symplex® F (Standard Process): Female Protomorphogen™ extract support for the pituitary, thyroid, adrenal glands, and ovaries.

Dosage: One to two tablets, three times per day with meals.

Symplex® M (Standard Process): Male Protomorphogen™ extract support for the pituitary, thyroid, adrenal glands, and testicles.

Dosage: One to two tablets, three times per day with meals.

Paraplex® (Standard Process): Pituitary, thyroid, adrenal, and pancreatic Protomorphogen™ extract support.

Dosage: One to two tablets, three times per day with meals.

Primary Support: Adrenal Glands

Drenatrophin PMG® (Standard Process): Adrenal Protomorphogen™ extract support.

Dosage: One to two tablets, three times per day with meals.

Drenamin® (Standard Process): Adrenal Protomorphogen™ extract support along with Cataplex® G and Cataplex® C.

Dosage: Two to three tablets, three times per day with meals.

Symplex® F (Standard Process): Female Protomorphogen™ extract support for the pituitary, thyroid, adrenal glands, and ovaries.

Dosage: One to two tablets, three times per day with meals.

Symplex® M (Standard Process): Male Protomorphogen™ extract support for the pituitary, thyroid, adrenal glands, and testicles.

Dosage: One to two tablets, three times per day with meals.

Primary Support: Thyroid

Thytrophin PMG® (Standard Process): Thyroid Protomorphogen™ extract support.

Dosage: One to two tablets, three times per day with meals.

Symplex® F (Standard Process): Female Protomorphogen™ extract support for the pituitary, thyroid, adrenal glands, and ovaries.

Dosage: One to two tablets, three times per day with meals.

General Endocrine Support

Symplex® M (Standard Process): Male Protomorphogen™ extract support for the pituitary, thyroid, adrenal glands, and testicles.

Dosage: One to two tablets, three times per day with meals.

Primary Support: Ovaries

Ovatrophin PMG® (Standard Process): Ovary Protomorphogen™ extract support.

Dosage: One to two tablets, three times per day with meals.

Ovex® or Ovex® P (Standard Process): Ovarian Cytosol™ extract support.

Dosage: One to two tablets, three times per day.

Symplex® F (Standard Process): Female Protomorphogen™ extract support for the pituitary, thyroid, adrenal glands, and ovaries.

Dosage: One to two tablets, three times per day with meals.

Primary Support: Uterus

Utrophin PMG® (Standard Process): Uterine Protomorphogen™ extract support.

Dosage: One to two tablets, three times per day with meals.

Primary Support: Testes

Orchic PMG® (Standard Process): Testicle Protomorphogen™ extract support.

Dosage: One to two tablets, three times per day with meals.

Orchex® (Standard Process): Testicle Cytosol™ extract support.

Dosage: One to two tablets, three times per day with meals.

Symplex® M (Standard Process): Male Protomorphogen™ extract support for the pituitary, thyroid, adrenal glands, and testicles.

Dosage: One to two tablets, three times per day with meals.

Primary Support: Parathyroid

Cal-Ma Plus® (Standard Process): Parathyroid Protomorphogen™ extract support with calcium and magnesium.

Dosage: One to two tablets, three times per day with meals.

Primary Support: Pancreas

Pancreatrophin PMG® (Standard Process): Pancreatic Protomorphogen™ extract support.

Dosage: One to two tablets, three times per day with meals.

Paraplex® (Standard Process): Pituitary, thyroid, adrenal, and pancreatic Protomorphogen™ extract support.

Dosage: One to two tablets, three times per day with meals.

General Kidney Support

Defined

The kidneys are paired organs situated at the back of the abdomen, below the diaphragm, on each side of the spine. These two organs filter the blood thus excreting the end-products of metabolism in the form of urine, and regulate the concentration of sodium, hydrogen, phosphate, potassium, and other ions in the extracellular fluid.

Biological Functions of the Kidneys

Cardiovascular System

- The kidneys assist in regulating blood pressure.
- Erythropoietin, the hormone which controls the red blood synthesis, is produced in the kidneys.

Excretory System

- Approximately 25% of the blood pumped by the heart each minute is filtered by the kidneys, and toxins are excreted from the body via this filtration mechanism in the form of urine.
- The kidneys are responsible for excreting, nitrogenous waste products (ammonia), excess sodium, aluminum, urea, excess water and uric acid.
- The kidneys are responsible for the continual production of urine.

Metabolism

- The kidneys manufacture some endogenous creatine.
- The active endogenous form of vitamin D (1-25-dihydroxycholecalciferol) is manufactured within the kidneys from its precursor – 25-hydroxycholecalciferol.

Water & Water Balance

- The kidneys are the primary organs responsible for maintaining the balance of water within the body.

Supplementation

The following list of products provides those nutrients needed to maintain the healthy functioning of the kidneys.

Choose from any combination of the following products; however, consider using Renafood® as a primary, and then add others as the case dictates.

Renafood® (Standard Process): Desiccated kidney, tillandsia, kidney Protomorphogen™ extracts, carrot powder, vitamin A esters, wheat germ, oat flour, beet root, and kidney bean extract all of which supply the factors that are needed to support optimal kidney tissue regeneration and cellular functioning.

Dosage: Two to three tablets, three times per day with meals.

Cataplex® A (Standard Process): Provides not only the vitamin A complex but the associated fat soluble vitamins, trace minerals, and water soluble vitamin complexes that work synergistically with vitamin A for optimal healing of kidney tissue.

Dosage: Two tablets, three times per day with meals.

General Kidney Support

Chlorophyll Complex™ (Standard Process): The kidneys are composed largely of fat, thus, it would be wise to supply them with a rich source of fat-soluble vitamins. This is a fat soluble chlorophyll extract which is the form of chlorophyll found in green plants thus making it an excellent source of the fat-soluble vitamins.

Dosage: One to two perles, three times per day with meals.

Renatrophin PMG® (Standard Process): Kidney Protomorphogen™ extract support. This is also contained in Renafood®, however the case may warrant additional support.

Dosage: If used in conjunction with Renafood®, one tablet, three times per day.
    If used without Renafood®, two tablets, three times per day.

Arginex® (Standard Process): The last step in the conversion of ammonia to urea occurs when arginine is cleaved by arginase to produce urea and ornithine. Arginex® is a source of arginase. Arginase also has a role in the kidney's processing of ammonia produced from their utilization of glutamine and alanine.

Dosage: One to two tablets, three times per day.

Albaplex® (Standard Process): A combination formula of various individual Standard Process products, including Betacol®, Renafood®, Choline, Cataplex® A-C, Arginex®, Renatrophin PMG®, and Thymex®. This is intended as broad-based kidney support along with liver and immune support.

Dosage: Two to three capsules, three times per day with meals.

Rehmannia 1:2 (MediHerb): Kidney tonic.

Dosage: Four mL one to two times per day.

General Liver Support

The liver is truly a remarkable organ and is capable of a great variety of functions. A complete review of its functions are beyond the scope of this text, but it would be fair to say that it is either directly or indirectly involved with every physiologic and/or biochemical process in the body. However, some of the basic biological functions or systems that the liver is involved in are: cardiovascular system, detoxification, excretion, and metabolism.

Cardiovascular System

- The liver processes approximately three pints of blood every minute.
- The liver stores blood and filters blood by removing infectious organisms.
- Blood arrives at the liver from two sources: from the intestines via the portal vein carrying dietary nutrients and dietary toxins and via the hepatic artery.

Detoxification

The liver is the chief organ of detoxification of toxic chemicals that enter the body.

- Phase I enzymes in the liver neutralize many toxic chemicals or convert them to primary metabolites. These metabolites are more toxic than their precursor toxins. This process of detoxification is known as the phase I cytochrome P-450 and phase II detoxification system.
- It is the role of phase II enzymes in the liver to process the primary metabolites of toxins produced by phase I enzymes.

Excretory System

- The liver is in involved in the urea cycle which involves the conversion of ammonia (derived from nitrogen from amino acids) to urea.
- The liver clears the body of bilirubin, the yellow pigment produced when red blood cells die.

Metabolism

- Ingested alcohol is metabolized by the liver.
- The conversion of stored glycogen into glucose for release into the bloodstream occurs in the liver.
- The liver is responsible for converting fatty acids to ketone bodies via beta-oxidation.
- The liver is responsible for approximately twenty-five percent of basal metabolism.

The following substances are manufactured, stored, or metabolized in the liver: amino acids, carbohydrates, carotenoids, digestive enzymes, enzymes, hormones, ketones, minerals, phospholipids, proteins, quinones, sterols, and vitamins.

Amino Acids

- The non-essential amino acids are manufactured within the liver.
- The conversion of glucogenic amino acids to glucose occurs in the liver.
- Glycine is manufactured within the liver from the lipotrophic factor, choline.
- Tryptophan is stored in large quantities within the liver.
- S-Adenosylmethionine (SAM) is concentrated and produced in the liver.

Carbohydrates

- Galactose and fructose are converted into glucose in the liver.
- Glucose is converted into fat in the liver.
- Heparin is manufactured within the liver.

Carotenoids

- Beta carotene and lycopene are stored in the liver.

General Liver Support

Digestive Enzymes

- The liver manufactures bile.

Enzymes

- Acetylcholinesterase is synthesized by the liver.

Hormones

- Approximately 80% of the conversion of T4 to T3 occurs in the liver.

Ketones

- Acetone is manufactured in the liver as a byproduct of the metabolism of fatty acids for excretion via the urine or released in the breath.
- Beta-hydroxybutyric acid and acetoacetic acid are manufactured in the liver as byproducts of the metabolism of fatty acids for cellular fuel or excretion via the urine.

Minerals

- Cobalt and approximately 15% of the body's copper concentrates in the liver.
- The liver stores ferritin (the endogenous storage form of iron).
- Manganese accumulates in the liver.

Phospholipids

- Endogenous phospholipids are produced by the liver.

Proteins

- Synthesis of endogenous proteins occurs in the liver.
- The liver manufactures lipoproteins.
- The liver can convert proteins to fat.

Quinones

- The liver contains high concentrations of Coenzyme Q10.

Sterols

- Cholesterol is produced by the liver.

Vitamins

- The liver has the capacity to store approximately a six to nine month supply of folic acid in its methyl folate form.
- The liver stores vitamin A as retinyl esters (i.e. combined with a fatty acid, usually as retinyl palmitate).
  Note: Liver malfunction can interfere with the metabolism of vitamin A.
- Vitamin B1and vitamin E are found in high concentrations in the liver.
- Vitamins C, K, B2, B5, B6, B12, and biotin are stored in the liver.
- Vitamin D is stored in the liver as 25-hydroxycholecalciferol which is the (endogenous) form of vitamin D manufactured within the liver from cholecalciferol (vitamin D3).

Supplementation

With all the important roles that this organ performs, it must be supplied with a constant source of nutrients to support optimal cellular functioning. The following list of products provide those nutrients needed at a cellular level to help support optimal hepatocyte and Kupffer cell functions.

Primary Support

Choose from any combination of the following products; however, consider using **Livaplex®** as a base product, then add others as the case dictates.

General Liver Support

Livaplex® (Standard Process): The combined action of A-F Betafood®, Betacol®, Antronex®, Spanish Black Radish, Chezyn®, and Hepatrophin PMG® provides the factors that are needed to support healthy bile production and flow, bowel detoxification, liver decongestion through the use of to lipotrophic factors, hepatic Protomorphogen™ extract support, and enhanced blood flow through the portal vein.

Dosage: Two to three capsules, three times per day with meals.

A-F Betafood® or Betafood® (both Standard Process): A-F Betafood® supports bile production and flow through the use of various food factors; Betafood®, however, is more bile thinning because it contains a higher concentration of beet root and beet leaves, which make it higher in betaine - the bile thinning factor that also gives beets their red color.

Dosage: A-F Betafood® – Six to nine tablets per day with the dosage divided between three meals.
   Or
Betafood® – Three to six tablets per day with the dosage divided between three meals.

Hepatrophin PMG® (Standard Process): Liver Protomorphogen™ extract support.

Dosage: One to two tablets, three times per day with meals.

Cataplex® G (Standard Process): Provides the B vitamin complex factors with the greatest ability to support hepatocellular regeneration.

Dosage: Two tablets, three times per day with meals.

Super-Eff®: Since the liver is one of the largest "consumers" of fatty acids in the body, it is important that it be supplied with a good supply of essential fatty acids. Super-Eff provides the fatty acids in a form that would naturally occur after healthy hepatic tissue normally processes fats. You could say the Super-Eff® is a more advanced form of fats which supplies the hepatic tissue what it needs without having to go through processing the fat itself.

Dosage: Two tablets, three times per day with meals.

Chlorophyll Complex™ (Standard Process): This is chlorophyll in its natural form. It is not a dry powder, which makes it an excellent source of the fat soluble vitamins of which the liver has a high affinity for.

Dosage: One to two perles, three times per day with meals.

Betacol® (Standard Process): Consider this product when you suspect excess fat deposits in the liver. Betacol® supplies lipotropic factors to help move fat out of the liver and supports bile production and flow. It is also a source of methyl donors, thus supporting liver detoxification processes.

Dosage: One to two tablets, three times per day with meals.

OPC Synergy™ (Standard Process): Containing Masquelier's Original OPC antioxidant formula, OPC Synergy combines grape seed extract, buckwheat, red wine extract, green tea extract, and bilberry to provide important antioxidant support to the hepatic tissue. During normal cytochrome P450 phase I and phase II mechanisms, free radical production can result in hepatocellular damage if the tissues are not supplied with a steady influx of antioxidants.

Dosage: One tablet, two times per day with meals.

Silymarin (MediHerb): Hepatotrophorestorative, hepatoprotective, and choleretic.

Dosage: One tablet three to four times per day.

Heart Failure

Defined

Heart failure is not that the heart has stopped working; it is the inability of the heart to pump adequate amounts of blood to meet the metabolic needs of the body. Heart failure will result in poor tissue perfusion and increased interstitial volume.

Signs and Symptoms

Heart failure can be classified according to the side of the heart affected.

Left sided heart failure:

- Orthopnea, dyspnea, paroxysmal dyspnea
- Pale, cool skin
- Tachycardia
- Hemoptoysis
- Nonproductive cough
- Fatigue

Right sided heart failure:

- Right upper quadrant pain
- Jugular venous distention
- Hepatomegaly
- Nocturia
- Anorexia, nausea, and fullness
- Weight gain
- Ascites, edema or anasarca

Etiology

Heart failure may be found in conjunction with any of the following:

- Ischemic heart disease, generally due to coronary artery disease
- Hypertension
- Congenital defects (muscle, valves)
- Nutritional deficiency
- Damaging dietary fats (The majority of dietary fats bypass the portal system and are absorbed directly into the lymphatic system. The result is that the heart is exposed to these fats prior to being processed by the liver)
- Rheumatic heart disease
- Myocarditis
- Pregnancy
- Diabetes
- Hyperthyroidism
- Obesity
- Alcoholism
- Chronic lung disease
- Previous myocardial infarction

Treatment Considerations

- Provide nutritional components that support optimal energy production at the cellular level and maximize blood flow to bring oxygen and nutrients to the cardiac tissue.
- Utilization of heart Protomorphogen™ extracts
- Use of potassium sparing diuretics to enhance the removal of excess fluid accumulation
- Support optimal cardiac electrical activity

Heart Failure

Supplementation

Primary Support

Vasculin® (Standard Process): Provides the following:

- The B vitamins (Cataplex® B) needed for optimal cardiac deplorization and replolarization along with ATP production via glycolysis, the Kreb's cycle, and the electron transport chain.
- Source of the vitamin C complex (Cataplex® C), which will support the adrenal glands (backups to the heart) and enhance the blood's ability to deliver oxygen to the cardiac muscle.
- Support for the heart via Protomorphogen™ extracts.
- Source of the vitamin E complex (Cataplex® E), which provides protection against oxidative stress from free radicals. It reduces the aggregation of platelets and prevents oxidation of low-density lipoprotein cholesterol.

Dosage: Three tablets, three times per day with meals.

Cataplex® E2 (Standard Process): Specific fraction of the vitamin E complex that maximizes the delivery of oxygen to the cells.

Dosage: Two to three tablets, three times per day with meals.

Hawthorn (MediHerb): Hawthorn has been traditionally used for its cardiotonic, cardioprotective, hypotensive, antiarrhythmic, antioxidant, and vasodilatory effects.

Dosage: One tablet, three to four times per day.

Magnesium Lactate (Standard Process): Magnesium is essential for the cardiac muscle to release energy at the cellular level and for its vasorelaxant effects.

Dosage: One to two capsules, three times per day with meals.

Secondary Support: As Indicated

Dandelion Leaves 1:1 (MediHerb): Natural diuretic which is very high in potassium.

Dosage: Five mL, twice per day for edema.

Korean Ginseng 1:2 (MediHerb): Whole system tonic that increases oxygen carrying capacity of the red blood cells.

Dosage: Two and one half mL once or twice a day.

Hemorrhoids

Defined

Varicosities in the superior or inferior hemorrhoidal venous plexus. Enlargement and dilation of the plexus of superior hemorrhoidal veins above the dentate line cause internal hemorrhoids. Enlargement of the plexus of inferior hemorrhoidal veins below the dentate line results in external hemorrhoids, which may protrude from the rectum.

Signs and Symptoms

- Intermittent, painless bleeding during defecation
- Bright red blood on the toilet tissue or on the outside of the stool
- Anal itching along with vague anal discomfort
- Pain
- Secondary anemia

Etiology

- Constipation, low fiber diet, and straining at defecation
- Obesity
- Pregnancy
- Prolonged sitting
- Heavy lifting
- Liver disorders (e.g. liver cirrhosis, fatty liver) that can result in excessive venous pressure

Since the portal venous system contains no valves, factors that increase intravenous pressure in the perianal region can cause hemorrhoid formation. This includes factors which increase intrabdominal pressure such as pregnancy, coughing, defecation, coughing, sneezing, physical exertion, vomiting, and portal hypertension due to liver cirrhosis. Hemorrhoids are classified according to severity as follows:

- *First degree:* confined to the area around the anal canal.
- *Second degree:* prolapse occurs during straining but reduces spontaneously.
- *Third degree:* prolapse which requires manual reduction after each bowel movement.
- *Fourth degree:* hemorrhoids which are irreducible.

Treatment Considerations

- Improve venous tone, vein function, and venous return
- Enhance circulation
- For a congested liver that restricts the flow of blood from the portal vein, consider general liver support or hepatic detoxification.

Hemorrhoids

Supplementation

Primary Support

Collinsonia Root (Standard Process): Collinsonia root, also called Stone Root, has been used traditionally as a vascular astringent; helps maintain proper tone of the vascular system.

Dosage: Two to three capsules, twice daily with a full glass of water between meals.

Horsechestnut Complex (MediHerb): Combination of Horsechestnut, Butcher's Broom, and *Gingko biloba* which provides anti-inflammatory, venotonic, antioxidant, circulatory enhancement, collagen stabilizing, and vasoprotective properties.

Dosage: One tablet, two to three times per day.

Betacol® (Standard Process): Consider this product when you suspect excess fat deposits in the liver. Betacol® supplies lipotrophic factors to help move fat out of the liver and supports bile production and flow. It is also a source of methyl donors, thus supporting liver detoxification processes and liver decongestion.

Dosage: One to two tablets, three times per day with meals.

OPC Synergy™ (Standard Process): Containing Masquelier's Patented Original OPC antioxidant formula, OPC Synergy combines grape seed extract, buckwheat, red wine extract, green tea extract, and bilberry to provide oligoproanthocyanadins which improve microcirculation and provide additional venotonic, astringent, anti-inflammatory, and antioxidant support.

Dosage: One tablet, two times per day with meals.

Cataplex® A-C-P (Standard Process): Combination of the vitamin A and C complex factors along with the anti-capillary fragility factor named the vitamin P complex. These vitamin complexes are essential to maintain the integrity of the venous tissue.

Dosage: Two tablets three times per day with meals.

Hypercholesterolemia (Hyperlipoproteinemia)

Defined

Hypercholesterolemia is defined as abnormally high levels of cholesterol in the blood.

Hyperliproteinemia is an excess of lipoproteins in the blood due to a disorder of lipoprotein metabolism. The disorder may be acquired or familial.

- Acquired – occurs secondarily as a result of diet or some other disorder such as hypothyroidism, nephritic syndrome, or hypoadrenocorticism.
- Familial – inherited hyperlipoproteinemia.

Symptoms and Signs

Hypercholesterolemia initially is a silent disease with no outward symptoms until plaque formation in the arteries begins to affect circulation. Occasionally, when lipid levels are particularly high, fat may be deposited in the tendons and skin and forms bumps called xanthomas. Total blood cholesterol levels consist of several lipoproteins: VLDL's, LDL's, and HDL's. When determining health risk, it is more accurate to evaluate cholesterol levels by using various ratios of these lipoproteins versus using one measure alone.

Symptoms that may correlate with high lipid levels are:

- Peripheral artery disease
- Coronary artery disease
- Cerebrovascular disease
- Erectile dysfunction

- Enlargement of liver or spleen with resultant pancreatitis
- Angina due to coronary insufficiency
- Blood sugar imbalances

Etiology

Dietary cholesterol and saturated fat are the two main etiological factors often discussed when referring to elevated cholesterol and lipoprotein levels. These are important issues to concern ourselves with; however, we should also ask ourselves why the VLDL levels are high in the first place. To see why the liver would increase VLDL levels, we need to look at the following.

Excess glucose is stored as glycogen in the liver and skeletal muscles. Once glycogen stores are met, the liver converts excess glucose into triglycerides and cholesterol. These fats are then transported for storage by lipoproteins known as VLDL's and LDL's. The VLDL's transport cholesterol, triglycerides, and phospholipids from the liver to the peripheral tissues in order to avoid a build up of fat in the liver. Once the VLDL's have released their cholesterol, the lipoprotein is called an LDL, which consists mainly of triglycerides and phospholipids for deposition elsewhere in the body. HDL's are the lipoproteins that bring cholesterol back to the liver.

As can be seen from the previous explanation of lipoprotein synthesis, the typical American diet of excess consumption of refined carbohydrates will have an effect an elevating effect on lipid levels just based on the normal physiology of the body in response to high blood glucose.

In addition, the following are some of the other more common factors that may account for increasing lipid profiles:

- High saturated fat intake
- Excessive caffeine intake
- Hydrogenated fats (trans fats)
- Genetic predisposition (has a role in approximately one in five hundred people)
- Poor liver functioning
- Low thyroid function
- Poorly controlled diabetes

Hypercholesterolemia (Hyperlipoproteinemia)

- Obesity
- Reduced physical activity
- Insulin resistance
- Mental stress
- PCOS (Polycystic Ovarian Syndrome – a hormonal disorder characterized by multiple cysts in ovaries, irregular or no menstruation, obesity, and hirsutism)

Treatment Considerations

- Regulate hepatic cholesterol production
- Enhance bile production and flow
- Provide nutritional cardiovascular support

Supplementation

Primary Support

Garlic 5000mg (MediHerb): Hypocholesterolemic and blood thinning.

Dosage: One tablet, three times per day with meals.

Gastro-Fiber® (Standard Process): A combination fiber supplement. Fiber helps to reduce cholesterol in two ways:

1. The insoluble fiber feeds the microflora of the large intestine resulting in the liberation of short chain fatty acids such as butyrate, proprionate, acetate, and lactic acid. The acetate and proprionate are delivered to the liver where they have been shown to decrease the endogenous production of cholesterol and also have an effect on the liver's ability to handle glucose.
2. Soluble fiber will bind bile salts leaving less for reabsorption in the large intestine. Less reabsorption causes the body to use more of its own cholesterol to synthesize more bile acids resulting in a lowering of cholesterol levels.

Dosage: Three capsules, two to three times per day with meals.

Soy Bean Lecithin (Standard Process): Systemically acts as a fat emulsifier resulting in the removal of fat from the vasculature back into circulation. This can be of benefit with abnormal cholesterol deposits. Phosphatidylcholine, found in Soy Bean Lecithin is a major constituent of bile. Due to its bile thinning properties, phosphatidycholine helps to draw cholesterol out of the liver through the bile. Once the cholesterol reaches the large intestine the dietary fiber then can bind it up for removal via defecation.

Dosage: Three perles, three times per day with meals.

Note: When recommending Soy Bean Lecithin long term, add twelve Calcium Lactate (Standard Process) per day to the protocol. This is to avoid the possible removal of calcium from the bones to balance the phosphorous which is naturally present in Soy Bean Lecithin. For those with osteoporosis, consider Choline (Standard Process) at a dosage of two tablets three times per day instead of Soy Bean Lecithin. If using Choline, additional Calcium Lactate is not needed.

Cyruta® (Standard Process): Contains buckwheat leaf juice and seed extract along with inositol which support normalization of cholesterol and glucose levels.

Dosage: Two tablets, three times per day with meals.

Cholaplex® (Standard Process): Provides lipotrophic factors which support mobilization of fats from the peripheral tissues to the liver and the subsequent hepatic metabolism of blood fats.

Dosage: Three capsules, three times per day with meals.

Hypercholesterolemia (Hyperlipoproteinemia)

A-F Betafood® (Standard Process): Provides those nutrients needed to promote optimal hepatic production and flow of bile. Nearly all the cholesterol produced by liver is used for bile salt synthesis. In the large intestine the bile salts are absorbed by the dietary fiber and excreted.

Dosage: Two tablets, three times per day with meals.

Note: If there are no contraindications, then the Purification Program can be an excellent alternative to the above noted protocol regarding altering a lipid profile. Refer to the section titled *Detoxification* for more information.

Clinical Notes

Lifestyle Modification should be included when attempting to alter a lipid profile. Some basic modifications are as follows:

- Reduce saturated fat intake
- Increase fiber intake
- Increase consumption of oily fish (e.g. salmon, sardines)
- Increase consumption of the essential fatty acids such as flaxseed oil or a good quality fish oil.
- Aerobic exercise under the supervision of a clinician should be initiated
- Eliminate partially hydrogenated fats from the diet
- Reduce refined sugar and carbohydrate intake (this includes bagels, crackers, pasta, breads, cereals, etc.)

Hypoglycemia

Defined

An abnormally low concentration of glucose in the plasma that leads to symptoms of CNS dysfunction or sympathetic nervous system stimulation.

Signs and Symptoms

- Irritability
- Afternoon or mid-morning headaches
- Lethargy
- Anxiety
- Mental confusion
- Depression
- Weight gain
- Heart palpitations

- Excessive appetite
- Eat when nervous
- Hungry between meals
- Get shaky if hungry
- Elevated cholesterol levels
- Light headed if meals delayed
- Crave sweets or coffee in the afternoon

Etiology

Each patient may present with a variety of factors which influence blood sugar levels.

- Overeating of refined carbohydrates.
- Inadequate liver functioning (inability of hepatocytes to perform glycogenesis, gluconeogenesis, beta-oxidation, and deamination).
- Pancreatic fatigue (reduced insulin and/or glucagon production).
- Adrenal fatigue resulting in decreased cortisol and sympathetic hormone(s) production.
- Hypothyroidism
- Hypopituitism
- Nutritional deficiencies, especially the B vitamin factors which are critical to supporting ATP production at the cellular level.
- Overindulgence of unhealthy fats (refined oils, hydrogenated oils, trans fatty acids, rancid cooking oils) coupled with dietary lack of essential fatty acids (Omega 3 and Omega 6).
- Inherited hepatic enzyme deficiencies that restrict hepatic glucose release (e.g. glucose-6-phosphatase, phosphorylase, pyruvate carboxylase, fructose 1-6 diphosphatase, and glycogen synthetase).
- Alcohol abuse
- Inherited defects in fatty acid oxidation, including carnitine deficiency.
- Inherited defects in ketogenesis.
- Drugs (e.g. insulin, sulfonylureas, salicylates, propranolol, pentamidine, and disopyramide).
- Islet cell adenoma or carcinoma.
- Severe disease (e.g. viral hepatitis, cirrhosis, or cancer).
- Severe renal disease
- Insulin resistance
- Emotional and physical stress

Treatment Considerations

- Provide digestive enzymes to ensure optimal digestion of proteins, fats, and carbohydrates.
- Use of Protomorphogen™ extract support for the liver and pituitary gland.
- Adrenal support both nutritionally and with trophorestorative herbs.
- Nutritional support to facilitate hepatic handling of glucose and fatty acids.
- Use of remedies to counteract the effects of insulin resistance.
- Employ the benefits of antidiabetic and hypoglycemic herbs.

Hypoglycemia

Note: In order to obtain maximum stabilization of blood sugar, it is imperative that the patient makes the necessary lifestyle changes. Patients should be informed that without the appropriate dietary modifications supplementation alone may not produce the best results. For additional information regarding liver and adrenal gland support refer to the appropriate sections in this manual.

Supplementation

Primary Support

Diaplex® (Standard Process): A combination of various Standard Process product ingredients, as seen in parenthesis, that support carbohydrate handling as described below.

- Digestive support to enhance the breakdown of protein, carbohydrates, and fats in the stomach and small intestine (Zypan®).
- Supports the emulsification of fatty acids in the small intestine via providing those nutrients needed for adequate bile production and flow (A-F Betafood®).
- Decongests hepatic tissues through the use of lipotrophic agents (Betacol®).
- Protomorphogen™ extract support for the pancreas and pituitary glands. (Pancreatrophin PMG®, Pituitrophin PMG®).
- Enhances pancreatic function through the use of pancreatic Cytosol™ extracts.
  Note: There is no pancreas Cytosol™ extract available as a single product from Standard Process.
- A source of arginase (Arginex®). By supplying arginase, we are supporting urea production in the liver hence taking the stress off the kidneys. Arginase also has a role in the kidneys processing of the ammonia produced from their utilization of glutamine and alanine.

Dosage: Three tablets, three times per day with meals. Depending on the case, you may consider the addition of one or more of the individual products contained within Diaplex® at a dosage applicable to your particular case.

Note: For the vegetarian, consider **DiGest Phytosynergist™ or Digest tablets (MediHerb).** The combined action of the bitter herbs in this formula enhances hydrochloric acid production, bile release, and the release of pancreatic digestive enzymes into the gastrointestinal tract. This product should be taken at a dosage of five m,L fifteen to twenty minutes before each meal or one tablet, three times per day with meals.

Cataplex® GTF (Standard Process): GTF (Glucose Tolerance Factor). This unique product not only supplies chromium in a bioavailable form to improve cellular receptivity to insulin, but also adrenal, pancreatic, and liver support. Source of cysteine, a sulfur containing amino acid needed to form the disulfide bridge that links the two polypeptide chains of the protein insulin and supports cellular utilization of fatty acids for energy synthesis.

Dosage: One to two tablets, three times per day with meals.

Gymnema 4g or Gymnema 1:1 (both MediHerb): A bitter, antidiabetic, and hypoglycemic herb. Gymnema reduces the rate of absorption of simple sugars from the intestinal tract into the portal blood stream. The liquid has the additional benefit of helping to reduce the sense of taste for sweet foods.

Dosage: Gymnema 4g - One tablet, two times per day.
Or
Gymnema 1:1 – Four mL three times per day.

Hypothyroidism

Defined

An ailment characterized by underactivity of the thyroid gland resulting in insufficient production of thyroid hormones. Hypothyroidism is classified as primary hypothyroidism (disorder of the thyroid gland itself), secondary hypothyroidism (failure to stimulate normal thyroid function), or subclinical hypothyroidism (also called mild thyroid failure) which is a more common form of hypothyroidism, often with no or few symptoms.

Signs and Symptoms

Some of the more common symptoms include:

- Unexplained weight gain
- Cold intolerance
- Elevated cholesterol and triglyceride levels
- Increased capillary permeability and reduced lymphatic drainage which can result in edema
- Loss of libido
- Menstrual irregularities, typically menorrhagia
- Infertility
- Miscarriages, premature deliveries, and stillbirths are common
- Rough, dry skin
- Dry, course, brittle hair
- Hair loss
- Lateral part of the eyebrows falling out
- Nails can become brittle and will typically show transverse grooves
- Fatigue, depression, and weakness are some of the first symptoms to appear
- Difficulty concentrating and memory lapses
- Carotenemia
- Joint stiffness and muscular weakness
- Joint pain and tenderness
- Constipation
- Impaired kidney function
- Shortness of breath
- Periorbital edema
- Decreased cardiac output, slow pulse rate, congestive heart failure, signs of poor peripheral circulation
- Anorexia
- Absent Achilles reflex
- Abdominal distention
- Behavioral changes

Etiology

Primary hypothyroidism (disorder of the thyroid gland):

- Radiation therapy or thyroidectomy
- Inflammation, chronic autoimmune thryoiditis (Hashimoto's thyroiditis), or conditions such as sarcoidosis (rare) and amyloidosis

Secondary (failure to stimulate normal thyroid function):

- Inadequate conversion at the cellular level of T4 to T3 (this conversion mainly occurs in the liver and to a lessor extent in the kidneys)
- Inadequate production of thyroid hormone
- Inborn errors of thyroid hormone synthesis

Hypothyroidism

- Iodine deficiency
- Insufficient production of thyroid stimulating hormone (TSH) from the pituitary gland
- Use of antithyroid medications such as propylthiouracil
- Hypothalamic failure to produce (TRH) thryrotropin releasing hormone
- Exposure to environmental toxins
- Excessive consumption of fluoride
- Inadequate digestive processes resulting in mal-absorption of nutrients required for optimal thyroid function

Treatment Considerations

- Nutritional support to ensure optimal production of thyroid hormones.
- Those patients with an under-functioning thyroid gland may need to be on nutritional support long-term before a clinical judgment regarding the efficacy of support can be made. Keep in mind that if no significant improvement has been noticed and the patient is still not feeling well, then the appropriate referral should be considered. If the patient however opts to continue with natural support, supplementation should be continued for at least one year to see if a positive response can be achieved.
- For those patients who have been on thyroid medication, it may be difficult to restore thyroid function due to involution of the gland.

Supplementation

Primary Support

For Men

Thytrophin PMG® (Standard Process): Thyroid Protomorphogen™ extract support.

Dosage: One to two tablets, three times per day with meals.

Cataplex® F (Tablets) (Standard Process): Source of unsaturated fatty acids and 95 mcg of iodine per tablet. The fatty acids contained in this product are needed to ensure optimal delivery of iodine to the thyroid gland.

Dosage: One to two tablets, three times per day with meals.

For Women

Thytrophin PMG® (Standard Process): Thyroid Protomorphogen™ extract support.

Dosage: One to two tablets, three times per day with meals.

Cataplex® F (Perles) (Standard Process): Source of unsaturated fatty acids. The fatty acids contained in this product are needed to ensure optimal delivery of iodine to the thyroid gland.

Dosage: One to two perles, three times per day with meals.

Along with one of the following:

Trace Minerals-B12™ (Standard Process): Contains kelp, alfalfa, and other synergistic factors which make this a wonderful food delivery formula of trace minerals, while at the same time providing 145 mcg of iodine per tablet. Trace minerals are required cofactors for the enzyme iodothyronine iodinase, which is the enzyme that converts T4 to T3.

Dosage: One tablet, three times per day with meals.

Or

81

Hypothyroidism

Iodomere® (Standard Process): Combined actions of sea conch, iodine (200mcg per tablet), carrot powder, and liver powder make this a good source of essential and non-essential amino acids, while simultaneously providing additional factors needed to support optimal thyroid functioning.

Dosage: One tablet, one to three times per day with meals.

Secondary Support: As Indicated

Paraplex® (Standard Process): Pituitary, thyroid, adrenal, and pancreas support utilizing Protomorphogen™ extracts. This product provides broad-based endocrine support utilizing Protomorphogen™ extracts.

Dosage: Two tablets, three times per day with meals.

Eleuthero (MediHerb): An adaptogenic herb which helps increase the body's resistance to physical, emotional, biological, or environmental stressors and promotes normal physiologic function. Anyone with sub-optimal thyroid may benefit from the use of an adaptogenic herb.

Dosage: One tablet, three to four times per day.

Note: Consider the following functional test to evaluate thyroid activity, developed by Broda Barnes M. D.: At night, have the patient shake down a thermometer – be sure that it is shaken down and below 95 degrees. The next morning, upon awakening, have the patient put the thermometer under the arm with the bulb in the armpit with no clothing between it and the armpit, and leave it there for 10 minutes. After 10 minutes, they should take the thermometer out, read it, and write down the result right away. This is known as their Early AM Basal Temperature, and the "normal" should be between 97.8 and 98.2 degrees. This reading taken by armpit is somewhat lower and somewhat more accurate than by mouth. If the patient has a low-grade infection, the reading may be higher than their "normal". Therefore if it is outside that range above, they should repeat the above procedure every other day for a week or so. If the patient is a menstruating female, have her begin taking readings on the second and third day of her period.

Inadequate Liver and Gallbladder Functioning (Digestion)

Defined

In order to appreciate the importance of the liver and gallbladder regarding digestion, it is important to look at the role that bile plays in this multifaceted physiological event.

Bile is composed primarily of bile salts, cholesterol, phosphatidylcholine, and bilirubin. The contraction of the gallbladder to release its contents is triggered through a series of steps that commences with the introduction of food, especially fat and protein, into the duodenum. This triggers the release of secretin and cholecystokinin from the duodenum which in turn triggers the following to be released into the small intestine: bicarbonate from the liver and pancreas, pancreatic digestive enzymes, and bile from the contraction of the gallbladder.

Bile has a detergent-like action on fat and together with pancreatic lipase, the emulsification of large fat particles to microscopic particles occurs. These microscopic particles, which are composed of bile salts, transport the fat-soluble vitamins A, D, E, and K, fatty acids, phospholipids, and cholesterol. Once absorbed into the enterocytes of the small intestine, they make their way into the lymphatic vessels. From here, they are transported up the thoracic duct and into the subclavian vein.

Signs and Symptoms

- Fatty food intolerance
- Light colored stools
- Floating stools
- Pain between shoulder blades (especially right shoulder blade)
- Constipation
- Dry skin
- Halitosis
- Crave sweets
- Dairy products cause distress
- Itching skin and feet
- Dry hard stools
- History of gallbladder attacks

Etiology

The processed and adulterated foods in the American diet do not provide the precursor material needed to ensure optimal bile production and flow. Without these nutrients, healthy and abundant bile production is compromised.

Treatment Considerations

The goal of nutritional and/or herbal support is to provide those nutrients needed by the liver to ensure adequate bile production and proper flow.

Inadequate Liver and Gallbladder Functioning (Digestion)

Supplementation

Primary Support

Choose between option 1 or 2 for optimal primary support.

1. **A-F Betafood® (Standard Process):** A-F Betafood® supports bile production and flow through the use of various food factors.

   Dosage: Two to three tablets, three times per day with meals

2. **Livaplex® (Standard Process):** This formula is a combination of six individual Standard Process products which support the following actions: bile production and flow, bowel detoxification, liver decongestion due to lipotrophic factors, hepatic Protomorphogen™ extract support, and enhanced blood flow through the portal vein.

   Dosage: Two to three capsules, three times per day with food.

Secondary Support: As Indicated

Silymarin (MediHerb): Use if there is history of liver damage.

Dosage: One tablet, two to three times a day.

Livton® Complex (MediHerb): The herbs in this formula enhance bile production and flow. Livton Complex is not recommended for more than three months without taking a break from usage.

Dosage: One tablet, three times a day with meals.

Infections
(Bacterial and Viral)

Defined

Infectious diseases caused directly by infection by detrimental bacteria and viruses.

Signs and Symptoms

Acute inflammation is the body's response to cell injury or death. The chief signs of inflammation include:

- **Pain** – due to local pH changes, stimulation of pain receptors by tissue swelling, and chemicals excreted during the process of inflammation
- **Heat** – due to fluid leakage into the interstitial spaces, local vasodilatation, and increased blood flow to the area
- **Redness** – as a result of increased circulation and dilation of arterioles to the site
- **Swelling** (edema) – due to fluid leakage into interstitial spaces, local vasodilatation, and blocked lymphatic drainage

Fever

A fever typically follows the introduction of an infectious agent. A fever can help fight an infection because many microorganisms are unable to survive in this type of environment.

Leukocytosis

Leukocytosis is the bodies increased production of white blood cells in response to the introduction of pathogens. During the acute stage, neutrophil count increases. The bone marrow also begins to release immature leukocytes because the neutrophils cannot meet the body's demand for defensive cells. As the acute phase quiets down and the damaged tissue is isolated, the next stage of the inflammatory process takes place. This is called the cellular stage of inflammation. Monocytes, neutrophils, and macrophages begin the process of phagocytosis of bacteria and damaged tissue. Monocytes and neutrophils via chemotaxis are attracted to the site of infection; they identify the antigen and attach to it. They then engulf, degrade, and destroy the microorganism that carries the antigen on its surface. The macrophages, which are a mature monocyte, arrive at the site later and stay in the area of inflammation for a prolonged period. Macrophages are involved in other roles besides phagocytosis. They prepare and process the antigens for a cellular immune response and prepare the area for healing. An elevated monocyte count is typically common during the resolution of a chronic infection and any injury.

Chronic Inflammation

Chronic inflammation is any inflammatory process which lasts longer than two weeks. An unresolved infection or poorly healed wound can lead to a chronic infection. Chronic inflammation can lead to loss of tissue function and permanent scarring.

Etiology

Bacterial Infections

Bacteria are single celled organisms. Some live on the skin, in the mouth, in the airways, and in the genitourinary and digestive tracts of people and animals.

Bacteria are classified in several ways. One way is by their shape (e.g. spherical, rod-like, spiral, and helical). Another way is by their color after a specific stain is applied. Bacteria that stain blue are called gram-positive, whereas bacteria that stain pink are called gram-negative. Gram-negative and gram-positive bacterial differ in the type of infections they produce.

Gram-negative bacteria have a unique outer membrane which prevents many drugs from penetrating them. This makes gram-negative bacteria more resistant to antibiotics then gram-positive bacteria. The outer membranes of

Infections (Bacterial & Viral)

gram-negative bacteria are rich in lipopolysaccharides. When gram-negative bacteria enter the bloodstream, these lipopolysaccharides can trigger a drop in blood pressure and a high fever. It is for this reason that bacterial lipopolysaccharides are referred to as endotoxins. Gram-negative bacteria are able to exchange genetic material (DNA) with other strains of the same species and with different species. Thus, should gram-negative bacteria undergo a mutation (genetic change) that produces resistance to a particular antiobiotic and then share DNA with another strain of bacteria, the second strain will therefore become resistant as well.

Gram-positive bacteria are slower to develop antibiotic resistance. Some gram-positive bacteria (e.g. Clostridium botulism and Bacillus anthracis) produce toxins that can cause serious illness.

A third way of classifying bacteria is by their oxygen use. Bacteria that can live and grow in the presence of oxygen are called aerobes. Bacteria that can survive in low levels of oxygen, or are poisoned by oxygen are called anaerobes. Anaerobes thrive in areas with low oxygen levels such as the intestine, decaying tissue, and deep wounds. Hundreds of species of anaerobes normally inhabit and live harmlessly on the mucous membranes of the intestinal tract, lining of the mouth, and vagina. Most anaerobic infections are caused from the body's own pool of bacteria.

Anaerobic bacteria tend to invade the muscle and skin tissue that has been damaged by surgery or injury. Spontaneous infections can develop in those people who have weakened immune systems or cancer. Anaerobes can cause infections of the sinuses and middle ear.

Disease causing anaerobic bacteria includes Peptococci and Peptostreptococci which are part of the normal flora of the upper respiratory tract, mouth, and large intestine and clostridia (which reside in the intestinal tract of animals and humans, as well as in soil, decaying vegetation, and in the intestinal tract of humans). Other anaerobes include Actinomyces, Fusobacterium and Prevotella, all of which are part of the mouth normal flora and Bacterioides, which is part of the normal large bowel flora.

Viral Infections

A virus is smaller than a bacterium or fungus and must invade a living cell to replicate. A virus can attach itself to a cell, enter it, and release its DNA or RNA inside of the cell. The viral genetic code takes control of the cell thus forcing it to replicate the virus. The infected cell usually dies because the virus inhibits it from performing its normal functions. Before the cell dies, however, it releases new viruses, which go and infect other cells.

Not all viruses kill the cells they infect; instead, they alter the cell's functions. At times the infected cell loses control over normal cell division and becomes cancerous. Some of the viruses that do not kill the cells they infect will leave their genetic material in the host cell. Here it remains dormant (latent infection) for an extended period. Should the cell become disturbed, the virus may be able to begin growing again and cause disease.

Viruses usually only infect one particular cell type.

Viruses can be transmitted in a variety of ways. Some can be swallowed, some may be inhaled, and some may be transmitted by the bites of insects such as ticks and mosquitoes.

Treatment Considerations

The following are some basic principles to consider when applying nutritional support and/or herbal remedies for an infectious microbe:

- Enhance immune function.
- Determine the source of the infection whenever possible. If the infection is identified as viral or bacterial, then more specific remedies can be recommended.
- Consider long term prophylaxis utilizing the appropriate remedies.

Note: Keep in mind that the immune system is an alliance of several organs and systems. In order for these systems to work adequately, the body must be supplied with macro and micronutrients so as to feed the body at the cellular level. Therefore, it is recommended that if herbal remedies are to be used, they are used in conjunction with the primary protocol.

Infections (Bacterial & Viral)

Primary Support

Calcium Lactate (Standard Process): Source of ionizable calcium for maintenance of tissue calcium levels. This is very important so as to support optimal white blood cell activity and ensure an optimal immune response.

Dosage: In the case of fever, two tablets every fifteen minutes until the fever drops. Once the acute symptoms subside, reduce the dosage to six per day for a minimum of two weeks. Best taken on an empty stomach.

Cataplex® C (Standard Process): Vitamin C complex with associated factors from alfalfa, mushrooms, buckwheat leaf, and bone marrow. The vitamin C complex has an important role in the defensive mechanism of the body and its need is increased when these defenses are being stressed (e.g. during fever, toxemia, and acute infections).

Dosage: In the case of fever, two tablets per hour until the fever has subsided. Once the fever has subsided, reduce the dosage to six per day for two weeks.

Note: As an alternative to Calcium Lactate and Cataplex® C, consider Congaplex® during the acute phase.

Congaplex® (Standard Process): Combination of the vitamin C and A complexes, thymus Cytosol™ extract, calcium lactate, and cellular protein precursor material in the form of RNA. This formula provides the immune system the nutrients needed to mount an efficient immune response.

Dosage: Adult – Four to six capsules, three times per day. Finish the bottle.
Child (less then 12 years old) – Two capsules, three times per day. Finish the bottle.

Note: Should it be desired to add herbal support to the above, then Echinacea Premium tablets or liquid should be considered as follows.

Echinacea Premium or Echinacea Premium Blend 1:2 (both MediHerb): Wonderful blend of *Echinacea angustifolia* and *Echinacea Purpurea*.

Dosage: **Echinacea Premium** – One tablet, three to four times per day.
In an acute situation, consider two tablets, three to four times per day for 24-48 hours and then reduce the dosage to three to four tablets per day.
Or
Echinacea Premium Blend 1:2 – Five mL, three to four times per day increasing to 5 mL six times per day in an acute condition and then reduce to five mL three times per day after 24-48 hours.

Secondary Support: As Indicated

Immuplex® (Standard Process): Provides the vitamin A, C, and E complexes, folic acid, cyanocobalamin, trace minerals, and liver, thymus, spleen, and bone Protomorphogen™ extracts along with other synergistic factors for optimal immune system support. This is not a product to be used for an acute case. It is recommended for patients with depleted immune systems and require those nutritional factors needed for long-term rebuilding and to optimize the immune response.

Dosage: Two capsules, three times per day with meals.

Andrographis Complex (MediHerb): Combination of Andrographis, *Echinacea angustifolia*, and Holy Basil. This formula is immune enhancing and can be especially useful for those suffering from an upper respiratory tract infection in conjunction with products noted under the primary protocol.

Dosage: One tablet, three to four times per day. Consider increasing the dosage to two tablets four times per day in an acute condition. Finish the entire bottle.

Infections (Bacterial & Viral)

St John's Wort 1.8g: Anti-viral specifically for enveloped viruses (see chart).

Dosage: One tablet, three to four times per day. For acute conditions such as shingles or herpes, consider two tablets four times per day until the acute episode is over.

Some common enveloped viruses:

Virus Family	Specific Virus	Conditions
Herpes viruses	Simplex Varicella Zoster Cytomegalovirus Epstein-Barr	Oral, genital, ocular Chickenpox Shingles Salivary gland disease Mononucleosis
Hepatitis	B, C, and D	Jaundice
Poxviruses	Vaccinia Variola Molluscum contagiosum	Mild pox disease Smallpox Epithelial lesions
Togaviruses	Rubella virus Alpha virus Flavivirus Ross River	German Measles Encephalitis Yellow fever Dengue fever Encephalitis Polyarthritis
Orthomyxoviruses	Influenza A, B, and C	Influenza
Paramyxoviruses	Paramyxovirus Mobilivirus Rubulavirus Pneumovirus	Parainfluenza 1-4 Measles Mumps Respiratory syncytial disease
Retroviruses	HIV	AIDS
Coronaviruses		Common Cold
Arenaviruses	Lymphocytic Choriomeningitic virus Lassa virus	Lymphocytic Choriomeningitis Lassa fever
Bunyaviruses	California virus	Enchepalitis
Rhabdovirus		Rabies

Insufficient Digestion: Parotid Gland, Stomach, Liver and Pancreas

Defined

Insufficient digestive function of the upper gastrointestinal tract as a result of poor parotid gland(s), salivary gland(s), stomach, liver/gallbladder, and/or pancreas secretions. Either one or any combination of these areas may be compromised in any one patient.

Signs and Symptoms

- Loss of taste for meat
- Large amount of foul smelling bowel gas
- Coated tongue
- Reflux/GERD
- Nausea
- Food intolerances and/or allergies
- Abdominal pain
- Anemia
- Diarrhea
- Indigestion ½ to 1 hour after eating
- Stomach bloating after eating
- Upper digestive gas, belching
- Fatty food intolerance
- Intestinal dysbiosis
- Nutrient deficiencies
- Anorexia
- Undigested food in stools
- Migraine headaches
- Constipation

Etiology

Digestive secretions appears to decline with age and may also be attributed to overeating and the chronic consumption of overly processed, enzyme deficient, synthetically manufactured, and nutrient depleted foods.

Treatment Considerations

1. Address primary discomforts
2. Improve gastric digestive function
3. Enhance bile production and flow
4. Facilitate pancreatic exocrine functioning

Depending on the individual, more than one or all of the above may need to be addressed.

Supplementation

Primary Support: Parotid Gland

Parotid PMG® (Standard Process): Parotid gland support utilizing parotid Protomorphogen™ extracts. The parotid gland has an important role in digestion and immune function in that it produces alpha amylase and antibacterial factors such as lysozyme, Immunoglobin A, and lactoferrin.

Dosage: One to two tablets, three times per day with meals.

Insufficent Digestion: Parotid Gland, Stomach, Liver, and Pancreas

Primary Support

To improve gastric and small intestinal digestive functioning, consider the following products.

Zypan® (Standard Process): Provides betaine hydrochloride, pepsin, and ammonium chloride along with pancreatic enzymes to support optimal protein, fat, and carbohydrate digestion. Consider this the chief Standard Process proteolytic product with some broad-based small intestinal digestive support added.

Dosage: One to two tablets per meal. Can be used long term. Contraindicated if an active ulcerative lesion is present.

Multizyme® (Standard Process): Provides enzymatic support for protein, fat, and starch digestion. This is a good alternative to Zypan® when additional acidity is contraindicated in the gastric region. *Both Multizyme® and Zypan® can be used simultaneously if so desired.*

Dosage: Two capsules, three times per day with meals. Can be used long term.

DiGest Phytosynergist™ (MediHerb): The combined action of the bitter herbs in this formula stimulates optimal secretion of saliva, hydrochloric acid, bile, and pancreatic digestive enzymes.

Dosage: Five mL, 15-20 minutes before each meal.

Note: DiGest Phytosynergist™ is an excellent alternative to Zypan® for those who are vegetarians, and prefer the use of an herbal bitter tonic.

Note: To improve hepatic bile production and flow, refer to section titled *Inadequate Liver and Gallbladder Functioning (Digestion).*

Irritable Bowel Syndrome (IBS)

Defined

Also referred to as spastic colitis or spastic colon, Irritable Bowel Syndrome (IBS) is a motility disorder involving the entire colon, causing recurring upper and lower gastrointestinal symptoms. It is a benign condition that has no anatomical abnormality or inflammatory component.

Signs and Symptoms

- Crampy lower abdominal pain which typically occurs during the day and is relieved by defecation or passage of flatus
- Abdominal distension and bloating
- Constipation that alternates with diarrhea, with one being dominant

- Nausea, vomiting
- Passage of mucus through the rectum
- Fatigue
- Painful bowel movements
- Full sensation even after a small meal

Two major clinical types of IBS have been described:

1. **Constipation-predominant IBS:** Constipation is common, but there is a variation of bowel movements. The majority of patients have pain over at least one area of the colon which is associated with periodic constipation alternating with a more normal bowel movement frequency. The stool will often contain clear or white mucus. Pain is either colicky, occurring in bouts, or a continuous dull ache which may be relieved with a bowel movement. Eating typically triggers symptoms. Bloating, nausea, flatulence, pyrosis, and dyspepsia can also occur.

2. **Diarrhea-predominant IBS:** Abrupt diarrhea that occurs immediately upon arising or during or immediately after eating. Nocturnal diarrhea is unusual. Bloating, pain, and rectal urgency are not uncommon, and incontinence may occur. Painless diarrhea is not typical and should lead the clinician to consider other diagnostic possibilities (e.g. osmotic diarrhea, malabsorption).

Etiology and Contributing Factors

In this disorder, the digestive tract is especially sensitive to many stimuli. Stress, diet, hormones, drugs, or minor irritants may cause the digestive tract to contract abnormally. The brain has immense control over the digestive system. Stress, anxiety, fear, depression, or any strong emotion can lead to constipation, diarrhea, and other changes in bowel function and can cause a flare-up of IBS. It is important to remember that the diagnosis of IBS can only be arrived at after other differential factors, such as, the following have been excluded.

- Excessive laxative use
- Lactose intolerance
- Cancer
- Candida albicans
- Parasites
- Infection
- Poor liver function
- Stress, anxiety, depression, and/or neurotic tendencies
- Hypersensitivity to gastrin and cholecystokinin

- Bowel disease
- Hyperthyroidism
- Insufficient digestive enzymes
- Food intolerance/allergies
- Insufficient dietary fiber
- High antibiotic use

Treatment Considerations

Since IBS is such a multifaceted condition, the individual patient's presentation needs to be taken into account. A thorough case history is imperative with IBS.

Irritable Bowel Syndrome (IBS)

Consider the following:

- Address abnormal bowel motility with the use of bowel relaxing remedies.
- Emotional overlays such as anxiety, depression, stress and Obsessive/Compulsive Disorder (OCD) may also be associated with IBS and should be considered as additional causative factors. Use of nervine tonics and adaptogens may be warranted.
- The typical American diet does not provide the nutrients that support optimal liver functioning. With poor liver function, insufficient bile production and flow will result.
- Bile is a natural laxative and plays a significant role in the maintenance of healthy bowel flora. Consider using whole food choleretics and/or cholagogues.
- Demulcent activity may be helpful.
- The use of bowel antiseptics may be warranted if bowel infection is suspected.
- Increase dietary fiber.
- Alteration of stool pH.
- Is the colon dysbiotic? Restoration of intestinal microflora may be required.
- Use of mucous membrane trophorestoratives may be warranted if this has been a long standing condition.

Supplementation

Primary Support

Cramplex (MediHerb): Helps ease intestinal spasm and pain associated with IBS.

Dosage: One tablet, three times per day.

Chamomile High Grade 1:2 (MediHerb): Provides carminative and spasmolytic activity.

Dosage: Four mL with water once per day.

Zymex® (Capsules) (Standard Process): Specialized yeast culture that supports the formation of lactic acid from carbohydrates in the large intestine which results in lowering the pH of the stool. Overall effect is to promote a healthy balance of intestinal flora.

Dosage: Two capsules, three times per day with meals.

Lact-Enz® (Standard Process): A probiotic manufactured utilizing a specific process that results in it not needing refrigeration. It is a source of *Lactobacillus acidophilus* and *Bifidobacterium longum* along with protease, amylase, lipase, and cellulose which help to maintain a healthy intestinal environment.

Dosage: Three capsules, two times per day at least one hour before or two hours after a meal is preferred. Taking the capsules away from the meals ensures maximum delivery of the probiotic into the small and large intestine.

Nevaton® (MediHerb): The combined action of Schisandra, St John's Wort, Damiana, and Skullcap help calm the nervous system, support bile production, and provide adaptogenic support.

Dosage: One tablet, three to four times per day.

Secondary Support: As indicated

Betafood® (Standard Process) and/or Livton® (MediHerb): If constipation is an issue, then consider supporting bile flow and production with these products.

Dosage: Betafood® – One to two tablets, three times per day with meals.
And/Or
Livton® – One tablet, three to four times per day with meals.

Note: Refer to section titled *Inadequate Liver and Gallbladder Functioning* for additional information regarding the above products and other choleretics and cholagogue-products.

Irritable Bowel Syndrome (IBS)

Gastro-Fiber® (Standard Process): Dietary fiber comes from the cellular walls of plants and has specific effects on different aspects of gastrointestinal function. Gastro-Fiber contains phytonutrients from psyllium, Collinsonia root, apple pectin, fennel seed, and fenugreek seed. These whole-food factors function synergistically to:

- Help cleanse and lubricate the intestines
- Encourage regular elimination
- Promote pH balance throughout the gastrointestinal tract
- Supports short chain fatty acid production

If lack of dietary fiber is an issue, the addition of this product in conjunction with dietary modification should be considered.

Dosage: Three capsules, three times per day with meals. Ensure adequate water intake.

Once the acute phase is under control, then restoring the integrity of the gut wall should be considered. The following formulas can be used as discrete formulas or in any combination based on the individual case.

Okra Pepsin E3 (Standard Process): Provides those factors needed for healing and restoration of the intestinal mucosal lining.

Dosage: Two to three capsules, three times per day between meals.

Aloe Vera 4.5:1 (MediHerb): The polysaccharides in aloe feed the microflora and aide in the restoration of the normal symbiotic microflora.

Dosage: Twenty-five mL, two to three times daily in water or juice. Best used for a minimum of three months for maximum clinical benefits.

Dermatrophin PMG® (Standard Process): Support for the epithelial tissues utilizing Protomorphogen™ extracts.

Dosage: One to two tablets, three times per day with meals.

Golden Seal 500mg (MediHerb): Mucosal membrane trophorestorative, vulnerary, antimicrobial and choleretic.

Dosage: One tablet, three times per day.

Clinical Observation

When addressing IBS, the etiology can be diverse and each case needs to be evaluated individually. For example, a patient with constipation will need to be treated differently than one suffering from diarrhea. The above noted products should be reviewed as to their roles in support of IBS and used in appropriate combinations.

Kidney Stones (Renal Calculi)

Defined

A kidney stone is a hard mass developed from crystals that precipitate from the urine and build up on the inner surfaces of the kidney. Stones can be found in the renal calyx, ureter, and the bladder.

Signs and Symptoms

- Sudden back pain localized in the back or flank in the area of the kidney. As the stone travels down the ureter, the pain pattern may move to the groin.
- Abdominal distention
- Nausea and/or vomiting
- Hematuria as the calculi abrade a ureter
- Chills and fever from infection

Etiology

The exact cause is unknown; however there are some common predisposing factors:

- Infection
- Dehydration
- Stasis in the urinary tract due to obstruction of urine flow
- Bone reabsorption due to immobilization
- Kidney disease
- Hyperparathyroidism
- Elevated uric acid
- Defective oxalate metabolism
- Urine pH changes

Most kidney stones form in adults between the ages of 20-40. Once a stone forms, there is a greater likelihood that additional stones will form. Therefore, knowing what kind of stone was passed is useful for prevention. Kidney stones can form from a number of different compounds. They are discussed here for reference:

- **Calcium Stones:** Approximately 85% of stones are composed predominantly of calcium compounds. The most common cause of calcium stone production is excess calcium in the urine (hypercalciuria). Calcium stones are composed of calcium that is chemically bound to oxalate (calcium oxalate) or phosphate (calcium phosphate). Of these, calcium oxalate is more common. Calcium phosphate stones typically occur in patients with metabolic or hormonal disorders such as hyperparathyroidism and renal tubular acidosis.

  Increased intestinal absorption of calcium (absorptive hypercalciuria), excessive hormone levels (hyperparathyroidism), and renal calcium leak (a kidney defect that causes excessive calcium to enter the urine) can cause hypercalciuria. Prolonged inactivity also increases urinary calcium and may cause stone formation.

  Renal tubular acidosis (inherited condition in which the kidneys are unable to excrete acid) significantly reduces urinary citrate and total acid levels which can lead to stone formation, usually calcium phosphate.

- **Uric Acid Stones:** The metabolism of protein produces uric acid. If the acid level in the urine is high or too much acid is excreted, the uric acid may not dissolve and uric acid stones may form. Genetics may play a role in the development of uric acid stones. Approximately 10% of patients with renal calculi will develop this type of stone.

- **Struvite Stones:** This type of stone, also called an infection stone, develops when a urinary tract infection (e.g. cystitis) affects the chemical balance of the urine. Bacteria in the urinary tract release chemicals that neutralize acid in the urine, which enables bacteria to grow more quickly and promotes struvite stone development. Struvite stones are more common in women because they have urinary tract infections more often. The stones usually develop as jagged structures called "staghorns" and can grow to be quite large.

Kidney Stones (Renal Calculi)

- **Cystine Stones:** Cystine is an amino acid that is not very soluble. Some people inherit a rare, congenital condition that results in large amounts of cystine in the urine.

Treatment Considerations

Since 85% of kidney stones are composed of calcium salts, the recommendations in this protocol are predominantly for stones that are small enough (under 5 mm) to pass safely. Large stones (over 1 cm) may require a different approach and will not be discussed here.

Supplementation

Nutritional and herbal recommendations should be considered as two phases. Phase I addresses the issue of the stone(s) and phase II pertains to healing and regeneration of renal tissue.

Primary Support: Phase I

Phosfood® Liquid (Standard Process): Source of ortho-phosphoric acid which reduces the pH of the urine. This reduction in pH can enhance the movement of calcium back into solution.

Dosage: Thirty drops (one dropper is equal to approximately ten drops), three times per day with a glass of water.

Cornsilk 1:1 or Marshmallow Root 1:5 Glycetract (both MediHerb): Demulcent herbs to reduce irritation in the ureters.

Dosage (for both): Two mL three times per day.

Note: Phase I should continue for at least two weeks. At which time if the clinician deems appropriate, proceed with phase II for at least twelve weeks.

Primary Support: Phase II

Renafood® (Standard Process): Desiccated kidney, tillandsia, kidney Protomorphogen™ extracts, carrot powder, vitamin A esters, wheat germ, oat flour, beet root, and kidney bean extract. Combined, these ingredients support optimal kidney tissue regeneration.

Dosage: Two to three tablets, three times per day with meals.

Cataplex® A (Standard Process): Provides not only vitamin A complex but the associated fat soluble vitamins, trace minerals, and water soluble vitamin complexes that work synergistically with vitamin A for optimal healing of kidney tissue.

Dosage: Two tablets, three times per day with meals.

Golden Seal 500mg (MediHerb): Golden Seal is a mucous membrane trophorestorative.

Dosage: One tablet, three times per day.

Clinical Note

- Instruct the patient to avoid the consumption of citrus juices, especially grapefruit, because of the net alkaline ash residue which has an alkalizing effect on the urine. The use of water or acid ash juice, such as unsweetened cherry or cranberry juice, should be recommended. Cranberry juice needs to be at least 27% pure cranberry juice to have a therapeutic effect.

- Ensure that the patient stays well hydrated.

Macular Degeneration

Defined

The macula is the region of the eye that is responsible for fine vision. Degeneration of this structure presents as two types: dry (atrophic) or wet (exudative).

Atrophic degeneration refers to a pigmentary disturbance in the macular region but no elevated macular scar, no hemorrhage, or exudation in the region of the macula.

Exudative degeneration refers to leaking fluid from the network of small capillaries which supply the eye close to the retina. Leaking and subsequent scarring of these vessels causes the loss of vision.

Signs and Symptoms

- As a result of neovascularization, there will be changes in central vision, such as a blank spot (scotoma) in the center of the page when reading.
- Straight lines appear distorted as a result of relocation of retinal receptors.

Etiology

Possible contributing factors:

- Free radical damage from smoking, bad fats, poor diet, etc.
- Compromised retinal circulation
- Hypertension
- Trauma
- Poor nutrition

Treatment Considerations

- Improve circulation
- Provide essential nutrients for nerve and blood vessel repair
- Antioxidant support
- Eye Protomorphogen™ extract support.

Supplementation

Primary Support

Oculotrophin PMG® (Standard Process): Protomorphogen™ extract support for the eye.

Dosage: One tablet, three times per day with meals. Start with one per day for one week, then two per day for one week, and then three per day. The dosage should be graduated so as to avoid any undue discomfort to the patient should a histamine reaction occur as a result of Protomorphogen™ extract use.

Bilberry 6000mg (MediHerb): Provides antioxidant, vasoprotective, and astringent support thus promoting integrity of the microvascular supply to the retina.

Dosage: One to two tablets, three times per day with meals.

Macular Degeneration

Cruciferous Complete™ (Standard Process): A combination of organically grown kale and Brussels sprouts which contain rich sources of lutein and zeaxanthin, two carotenoids that are deposited in the highest concentration in the region of the macula.

Dosage: Two capsules, three times per day with meals.

Cataplex® A-C (Standard Process): Source of the entire vitamin A and C complex which will support epithelial tissue regeneration.

Dosage: Two tablets, three times per day with meals.

Ginkgo 2000mg (MediHerb): Provides antioxidant support, improves the blood supply to the retina, and inhibits platelet aggregation.

Dosage: One tablet, three to four times per day with meals.

Note: This condition is the result of long-term oxidative damage at the cellular level along with compromised microvasculature. Supplementation should be considered for a minimum of 6-8 months.

Secondary Support: As Indicated

OPC Synergy™ (Standard Process): Additional astringent, vasoprotective, and antioxidant support. OPC Synergy™ contains grape seed extract (Masquelier's® patented Original OPC), red wine extract, green tea extract, bilberry, and buckwheat which makes this formula a rich source of antioxidants.

Dosage: One capsule, two to three times per day with meals.

Cataplex® E$_2$ (Standard Process): Supports optimal delivery of oxygen at a cellular level.

Dosage: One to two tablets, three times per day with meals.

Menopause

Defined

Menopause is the time in a woman's life when the ovaries stop producing an egg every four weeks and therefore menstruation ceases. *Climacteric* is a term that was used to describe the phase of irregular periods until complete cessation of menses. During the climacteric stage, menstruation usually decreases gradually, and the intervals between periods may lengthen. For some women, menopause may occur as a sudden cessation of menses. Menopause is a normal phenomenon and should be fairly asymptomatic.

Symptoms of Declining or Low Estrogen Levels

- A healthy menopause can be asymptomatic
- Hot flashes and sweating
- Fatigue
- Headaches
- Irritability
- Nervousness
- Sleep disruption
- Inability to concentrate
- Depression
- Anxiety
- Decrease in skin elasticity and tone
- Heart palpitations, tachycardia
- Recurrent urinary tract infections
- Recurrent vaginal infections
- Dry skin, eyes, and vaginal canal
- Decreased libido
- Memory loss
- Irregular cycles
- Menses can be heavy and/or more frequent
- Night sweats
- Nausea
- Constipation
- Diarrhea
- Arthralgia
- Myalgia
- Cold hands and feet

Etiology

Events and sequalae that occur during climacteric:

- FSH and LH are elevated in response to the reduced production of estrogen and progesterone by the ovaries
- Increased FSH can cause irregular cycles and irregular ovulation
- Estrogen levels can gradually or abruptly decrease as ovarian function declines
- All of the above may also result in lowered testosterone levels which can cause a drop in libido

Treatment Considerations

Clinically, it is sensible to address reduced estrogen levels, emotional complaints, and adrenal support first. After addressing these issues, consider the other symptoms related to menopause that are linked to a lowered quality of life.

Reduced Estrogen Levels

- Many menopausal symptoms are the result of the abrupt decline or irregular/diminished production of estrogen. Until the transition from ovarian production of estrogen to adrenal production of estrogen precursors takes place, the utilization of estrogen modulating herbs and adrenal nutrient support can reduce or eliminate symptoms associated with menopause.
- Support long-term estrogen production by providing ongoing adrenal support.

Menopause

Adrenal Support

- Continued adrenal support is necessary due to the role the adrenals play in forming the precursors that are converted to the steroid hormones during the menopausal years. If the adrenal glands cannot meet the increased demands placed on them during menopause, menopause can be more symptomatic.

Emotional Complaints

- Provide nutritional and herbal support to ameliorate depression, anxiety, loss of memory, and/or difficulty concentrating that may be present.

Supplementation

Primary Support

Important: If erratic periods or monthly menses are still occurring, add two Chaste Tree (MediHerb) every morning until menses ceases. This helps normalize ovulation and can be used for an extended period of time.

Reduced Estrogen Levels

The goal of herbal therapy is to ease the transition of lowering estrogen levels with the use of the following estrogen modulating products as single products or in a combination that is indicated for your particular case.

- **Wild Yam Complex (MediHerb):**

  Dosage: Six per day until discomforts subside, then three to four per day for maintenance.

  And/Or

- **Tribulus (MediHerb):**

  Dosage: Four per day until symptoms subside, then two per day for maintenance.

  And/Or

- **Black Cohosh (MediHerb):**

  Dosage: Three mL per day

Ovatrophin PMG® (Standard Process): Support for the ovaries utilizing *Protomorphogen*™ extracts.

Dosage: One to two tablets, three times per day with meals.

Adrenal Support

The following are two recommendations for supporting the adrenal glands. For those who prefer nutritional supplementation, utilize both Drenamin® and Cataplex® B. In those cases where herbal support is desired, utilization of both Rehmannia and Withania Complex as single formulas or in combination should be considered.

- **Drenamin® (Standard Process):** Provides adrenal *Protomorphogen*™ extract support along with the vitamin C complex and synergistic B vitamins to optimize adrenal function and responsiveness.

  Dosage: Two to three tablets, three times per day with meals.

- **Cataplex® B (Standard Process):** The B vitamins contained in this formula complement Drenamin® so as to supply all the B vitamins needed to ensure optimal ATP production at the cellular level. The thiamine in this formula is critical in order to facilitate the conversion of pyruvic acid to acetyl-CoA to support maximum ATP production in the mitochondria.

  Dosage: Two to three tablets, three times per day with meals.

Menopause

Note: Both Drenamin and Cataplex B can be used long term

Herbal Adrenal Support

- **Rehmannia Liquid (MediHerb):** Adrenal trophorestorative.

  Dosage: Four mL twice a day.

- **Withania Complex (MediHerb):** Contains *Withania somnifera* and licorice to provide adaptogenic support to the adrenal glands

  Dosage: One tablet, three to four times per day.

Emotional Support

The following MediHerb products can all be used long term.

- **Nevaton:** The combinations of herbs in this formula are beneficial for the symptoms of depression and anxiety.

  Dosage: One tablet, three to four times per day with meals.

- **St. John's Wort 1.8g:** For mild to moderate depression.

  Dosage: One tablet, three to four times per day.

- **Valerian Complex:** For those who suffer from a combination of anxiety, nervous irritability and insomnia.

  Dosage: One tablet, three to four times per day.

The period of climacteric can go on for years. Therefore, menopausal support may be indispensable for several years but not indefinitely.

Menorrhagia

Defined

Excessive bleeding that occurs during menses, either in number of days or amount of blood or both.

Signs and Symptoms

- Heavy bleeding with menses
- Fatigue

Etiology

- Endometriosis
- Uterine fibroids
- Infection
- Estrogen dominance

- Eicosanoid imbalance
- Endocrine disturbances
  (pituitary, thyroid, ovary, adrenal)

Other possible causes:

- Hypertension
- Diabetes mellitus
- Chronic nephritis

- Malposition of the uterus
- Adenomyosis of the uterus

Treatment Considerations

Treatment should be directed at reducing symptoms while determining if there is any underlying pathology.

Supplementation

Primary Protocol

Capsella Complex Phytosynergist™ (MediHerb): Consider this formula for heavy bleeding and the formula's hormone modulating and uterine astringent/tonic activity.

Dose: Five mL twice per day beginning three days before menses and increase during menstruation to five mL three to four times per day. Discontinue at the cessation of menses. This regimen can be used long term and should be continued every month. Allow at least 2-3 cycles to see maximum benefits.

Ovex® (Standard Process): Ovarian Cytosol™ extract.

Dosage: Two tablets, twice per day with meals.

Calcium Lactate (Standard Process): Ionizable calcium necessary to support blood coagulation.

Dosage: Two to four tablets, three times per day, preferably on an empty stomach.

Menorrhagia

Secondary Protocol: As Indicated

Chaste Tree (MediHerb): Supports proper ovulation by balancing the ratio of progesterone to estrogen during the luteal phase of the menstrual cycle.

Dosage: Two tablets once per day in the morning. With fibroids or endometriosis if you find that the symptoms have not improved as anticipated after eight weeks, then the dosage of Chaste Tree may need to be increased to four to six per day with the dosages divided up between the morning and evening.

Fe-Max Iron Tonic Phytosynergist™ (MediHerb): An herbal formula which supplies factors to support RBC blood production, promote vitality, support healthy digestion, and be a source of iron and B vitamins, including vitamin B12 and folic acid.

Dosage: Five mL three times per day with meals.

Wheat Germ Oil (Standard Process): A rich source of fat-soluble vitamins, such as vitamin A, E, F, and K. Wheat germ oil is helpful in reducing blood stagnation and clotting, reducing painful inflammations caused by leukotrine production from arachidonic acid, and enhancing oxygen delivery to the uterine tissue to help ease congestion.

Dosage: Two perles, three times per day with meals.

Clinical Notes

- *If menorrhagia is associated with uterine fibroids, infection, endometriosis, or premenstrual syndrome: Refer to the appropriate section of this text for more detailed information.*

- *Medical evaluation to rule out pathology should always be considered.*

Middle Ear Infection (Otitis Media)

Defined

Otitis media is an inflammation of the middle ear which can be suppurative, acute, persistent, unresponsive, or chronic. Otitis media is divided into two types of earache: acute otitis media and chronic or serous otitis media.

Acute otitis media is most common in children. It is important to remember that prolonged accumulation of fluid within the middle ear cavity will cause chronic otitis media and, possibly, perforation of the tympanic membrane.

Chronic suppurative otitis media can result in scarring, adhesions, and severe structural ear damage. Chronic secretory otitis media with the associated persistent inflammation and pressure may cause conductive hearing loss. Most frequent in children with tympanostomy tubes or those with a perforated tympanic membrane.

Recurrent otitis media is defined as the patient having three near acute otitis media episodes within six months or four episodes of acute otitis media within one year.

Otitis media with complications involves damage, such as retraction, adhesions, cholesteatoma, and intratemporal and intracrainial complications to middle ear structures.

Signs and Symptoms

Acute suppurative otitis media:

- Severe throbbing pain from pressure behind the tympanic membrane
- Symptoms of upper respiratory tract infection (coughing, sneezing)
- Hearing loss
- Mild to high fever
- Dizziness, tinnitus, vomiting, nausea
- Bulging, erythematous tympanic membrane; purulent drainage in the ear canal should the tympanic membrane rupture

Acute secretory otitis media:

- Sever conductive hearing loss which will vary depending on the thickness and amount of fluid in the middle ear cavity
- Popping, clicking sounds, or crackling on swallowing or with jaw movement
- Fullness sensation in the middle ear
- Echo during speech

Chronic otitis media:

- Scarring and thickening of the tympanic membrane
- Reduced or absent tympanic membrane mobility
- Formation of a cholesteatoma (a cyst-like mass in the middle ear)
- Purulent, painless discharge

Note: Should the tympanic membrane rupture, the patient may state that the pain has suddenly stopped. Complications that can arise may include abscesses (epidural, brain, and subperiosteal), jugular vein or sigmoid sinus thrombosis, meningitis, septicemia, facial paralysis, suppurative labyrinthitis, and otitis externa.

Etiology

Suppurative otitis media (bacterial infection):

- *Haemophilus influenzae,* most common cause in children under the age of 6
- Pneumococci

Middle Ear Infection (Otitis Media)

- *Moraxella catarrhalis*
- Staphylococci, most common cause in children 6 and older
- Beta-hemolytic streptococci
- Gram-negative bacteria

Chronic suppurative otitis media:

- Infection by resistant strains of bacteria
- Inadequate treatment of acute otitis episodes
- Tuberculosis (rare)

Secretory otitis media:

- Obstruction of the eustachian tube secondary to dysfunction of the eustachian tube from allergy or viral infection
- Barotrauma – pressure injury as a result of an inability to equalize pressures between the middle ear and environment:
  - during rapid underwater ascent in scuba diving (barotitis media)
  - during rapid descent of an aircraft in a person with an upper respiratory tract infection

Chronic secretory otitis media:

- Edema – chronic sinus infection, allergic rhinitis
- Mechanical obstruction – adenoidal overgrowth, tumors
- Inadequate treatment of acute suppurative otitis media

Treatment Considerations

- Provide immune support
- Promote drainage by addressing causative factors

Note: An ear infection is and can become very serious. The possibility of hearing loss is serious. When considering nutritional and herbal support for this condition with natural remedies, it may be wise to use natural remedies in addition to allopathic treatment for the acute case.

Supplementation

Primary Support: Suppurative Otitis Media

Choose from one or more of the following.

Echinacea Premium (MediHerb): For immune enhancement.

Dosage: Adult – One tablet, two to three times per day.
　　　　Children – Adjust dose accordingly.*

Thymex® (Standard Process): Thymus Cytosol™ extract.

Dosage: Adults – Two tablets, three times per day.
　　　　Children – One tablet, three times per day with meals. Consider mixing with applesauce if needed.

Congaplex® (Standard Process): This is to be used during the acute phase and not as a long term support product. The combination of the vitamin C and A complexes, thymus Cytosol™ extract, calcium lactate, and cellular protein precursor material in the form of RNA feed the immune system. The immune system utilizes the nutrients in increased amounts in order to mount an efficient immune response.

Dosage: Adult – Four to six capsules, three times per day. Finish the bottle.
　　　　Children – Two to four capsules, three times per day. Finish the bottle and consider mixing with applesauce if needed.

Middle Ear Infection (Otitis Media)

St John's Wort 1.8g (MediHerb): Anti-viral for enveloped viruses.

Dosage: Adults – One tablet, three times per day.
    Children – Adjust dose accordingly.*

Euphrasia Complex (MediHerb): For symptoms associated with allergies. Euphrasia Complex modulates mucus secretion, strengthens and tones the mucous membranes and provides immune support.

Dosage: Adults – Two to three, tablets three times per day.
    Children – Adjust the dosage accordingly.*

Primary Support: Chronic Suppurative Otitis Media

Echinacea Premium (MediHerb): Combination of *Echinacea angustifolia* and *Echinacea Purpurea* to enhance the immune response.

Dosage: Adults – One tablet, two to three times per day for adults.
    Children – Adjust dose accordingly.*

Immuplex® (Standard Process): Provides broad-based nutritional support to help ensure optimal immune functioning. Think of Immuplex® as Catalyn® for the immune system. It can be used long term.

Dosage: Adults – Two capsules, three times per day with meals.
    Children – One capsule, two to three times per day with meals.

St John's Wort 1.8g (MediHerb): Anti-viral for enveloped viruses.

Dosage: Adults – One tablet, three times per day.
    Children – Adjust the dosage accordingly.*

*Dosing Herbals for Children

Children who can swallow tablets

- Ages 12 and up get the adult dose
- Ages 6-12 half the adult dose
- Ages 6 and under one quarter adult dose

Children who can't swallow tablets

- Grind up tablets in an electric coffee grinder to provide the finest granulation method. The powder can then be added to applesauce or another food the child likes.

Migraine Headaches

Defined

A migraine is a headache that lasts four to seventy-two hours, is moderate to severe in intensity, is throbbing, and is unilateral. It is associated with vomiting, nausea, or sensitivity to smell, light, or sound and becomes worse with exertion

Signs and Symptoms

- Migraine can be preceded by a prodromal period of depression, irritability, and restlessness
- An aura which precedes the headache is transient and can include reversible neurologic, visual, and/or motor symptoms
- Visual aura which includes flashing lights, photophobia, and scintillating scotoma

- Nausea
- Vomiting
- Unilateral headaches which may not always occur on the same side
- Increased sensitivity to noise
- Diarrhea

Note: There is always the possibility that an intracranial pathology exists. Therefore, a conclusion of migraine is based on the symptom patterns when no such pathologies are present.

Etiology

The pathophysiology is not fully understood and the causes are unknown. Vascular changes occur in the brain and scalp arterial blood flow; however, it is unclear whether vasoconstriction and vasodilation are causes or effects of the migraine. Vasodilation is thought to activate pain receptors; however, this does not explain the complex changes in blood flow that occur in the brain during a migraine. In addition, there are a number of changes that occur in the nerve cells of the brain before the change in blood flow occurs. More than half of those who have migraines have a close relative who also experiences migraine headaches.

Some Common Triggers for Migraine Headaches

- Cycling estrogen (This is a major factor that may explain why the frequency is three times higher in females than in men. This may also explain why migraines are worse during puberty, premenopausal, and with those on oral contraceptives and estrogen replacement therapy.)
- Insomnia
- Hunger
- Stress
- Emotional issues
- Food intolerances
- Alcohol
- Hypoglycemia
- Helicobacter pylori infection

- Vertebral subluxation
- Cheese, red wine, and other vasoactive amines
- Toxins in the environment (perfumes, deodorants, colognes, cleaning products, etc.)
- Menses
- Toxins in the food (sulfites, coloring, preservatives, etc.)
- Bright lights
- Dairy
- Barometric changes
- Cerebral ischemia
- Blood viscosity, platelet aggregation
- Hypohydration

Treatment Considerations

When formulating a protocol, practitioners are advised to consider both the triggers and the symptoms to arrive at an optimal nutritional regimen. Below are some guidelines:

Migraine Headaches

- If the migraines occur premenstrually or with menses, refer to the appropriate sections in this manual
- Taking into account the inflammatory responses involved in these cases, the use of the appropriate remedies will be valuable as preventative agents
- For associated stress, depression, and/or anxiety refer to the appropriate sections in this manual
- If there is a correlation between the migraine and food, consider digestive support and/or liver support and then refer to the appropriate sections in this text as needed

Supplementation

Primary Support

Feverfew (MediHerb): Works well as a migraine prophylactic. Feverfew needs to be taken for four to six months in order to evaluate its effectiveness.

Dosage: One tablet, two times a day for four to six months. At which time, reduce the dose to one per day as the frequency of the migraines reduces.

Note: Feverfew (two tablets per day) can be combined with **Saligesic (MediHerb)** at a dosage of one tablet, two to three times per day for pain relief during a migraine episode.

Boswellia Complex (MediHerb): Provides modulation of the inflammatory response and aids in supporting the elimination of the end products of cellular metabolism that can contribute to inflammation.

Dosage: One tablet, two to three times per day.

Osteoarthritis

Defined

Osteoarthritis or degenerative joint disease is characterized by articular cartilage degeneration, synovial membrane changes, and underlying bone changes which are secondary. It is usually accompanied with pain and stiffness.

Signs and Symptoms

- Deep, aching joint pain
- Grating or crepitus of the joint during motion
- Stiffness in the morning and after exercise (relieved by rest)
- Altered gait from contractures
- Decreased range of motion
- Bony enlargements of distal interphalangeal joints (Herberden's nodes)
- Headaches (may be the direct result of cervical spine arthritis)
- Bony enlargement of proximal interphalangeal joint (Bouchard's nodes)

Etiology

Idiopathic – contributing factors:

- Genetic – reduced collagen synthesis
- Chemical – drugs that stimulate the collagen digesting enzymes such as corticosteroids in the synovial membranes
- Metabolic – endocrine disorders such as hyperparathyroidism
- Mechanical factors such as repeated stress, injury, and joint misalignment
- Poor diet and/or inadequate digestion
- Imbalance of the plasma calcium-phosphorous ratio

Secondary – identifiable predisposing event:

- Trauma (most common)
- Obesity, poor posture
- Congenital deformity
- Occupational stress

Treatment Considerations

- Provide nutrients needed to maintain healthy connective tissue
- Utilization of bone Protomorphogen™ extracts
- Use of alkalizing, depurative, anti-inflammatory, and circulatory stimulating herbs
- Consider systemic detoxification with the use of the Standard Process Purification Program

Note: It may not be possible to undue the degeneration that has already occurred, however nutritional support and lifestyle management should be suggested with the goal of reducing or halting any further progressive degenerative changes along with providing symptomatic relief.

Osteoarthritis

Supplementation

Primary Support

Boswellia Complex (MediHerb): The overall synergistic effects of the herbs in this formula reduce inflammation, facilitate the processing of metabolic acids, and improve joint circulation.

Dosage: Two tablets, twice per day.

Ostarplex® (Standard Process): Source of minerals, vitamins, mineral complexes, amino acids, bone Protomorphogen™ extract, and enzymes, all of which are needed in maintaining strong, healthy connective tissue. Source of lipotrophic and other factors to support hepatic detoxification mechanisms along with phosphoric acid to combat calcium deposits.

Dosage: Four capsules, three times per day with meals.

Glucosamine Synergy™ (Standard Process): Provides vitamins and minerals along with bone Protomorphogen™ extract support, essential fatty acids, vitamin D, and calcium lactate to support and maintain healthy bone and joints.

Dosage: One capsule, three times per day with meals.

Organically Bound Minerals (Standard Process): Provides alkaline ash minerals to combat excess acidity produced via the over consumption of refined products.

Dosage: One to three tablets, three times per day with meals.

Note: Iodine is contained within Organically Bound Minerals

Osteoporosis

Defined

A metabolic disorder in which the rate of bone resorption accelerates while the rate of bone formation slows, resulting in a loss of bone mass. Osteoporosis may be primary or secondary to an underlying disease.

Signs and Symptoms

- Typically osteoporosis is asymptomatic until a fracture occurs. Fractures can be spontaneous or secondary to trauma (a fall is usually the precipitating event) with the anterior thoracic crush-type vertebral fracture and hip fracture being the most common break sites.
- Progressive deformity (loss of height, deformity)
- Reduced exercise tolerance

Etiology

The mechanisms underlying the disparity in the rates of bone resorption and formation are complex and diverse and can be influenced by:

- Unknown factors
- Contributory factors such as:
    - declining adrenal and gonadol function
    - mild but prolonged negative calcium balance
    - estrogen deficiency
    - sedentary lifestyle
    - Liver and kidney insufficiency
    - Digestive insufficiency
- Prolonged corticosteroid, heparin, and anticonvulsant therapy
- Osteogenesis imperfecta
- Total immobilization or bone disuse
- Endocrine disorders such as hyperparathyroidism, hyperthyroidism, diabetes mellitus, Cushing syndrome
- Alcoholism, smoking, malabsorption, malnutrition
- Poor diet

Treatment Considerations

In addition to providing those nutritional factors needed to ensure optimal bone growth, you may need to consider some of the previously mentioned etiological links when working with your particular patient.

Supplementation

Primary Support

This protocol provides the nutrients needed to support optimal bone health and protect from bone loss.

Calcium Lactate (Standard Process): A balanced calcium and magnesium supplement in the proper 5:1 ratio. Calcium lactate is absorbed once ionized by the stomach acid.

Dosage: Four tablets, three times per day. Best taken away from meals.

Note: This is not a calcium meal replacement. The inclusion of this product is to supplement the diet with a readily available form of calcium while providing the associated synergistic cofactors required for bone mineralization.

110

Osteoporosis

Biost® (Standard Process): Bone Protomorphogen™ extract along with veal bone to supply those factors needed for bone growth and repair.

Dosage: Two tablets, three times per day with meals.

Calcifood® or Calcifood® Powder (both Standard Process): Both provide vitamins, minerals, enzymes, and amino acids needed for proper bone formation and maintenance. Source of heat labile amino acids.

Dosage: **Calcifood®** – Two wafers, three times per day with meals.
        Calcifood® Powder – One tablespoon, three times per day in juice or water.

Secondary Support: As Indicated

Catplex® D (Standard Process): Provides cholecalciferol (vitamin D3) which is normally formed in the skin by sunlight. Vitamin D works synergistically with the parathyroid glands,, liver, and kidneys to increase bloods calcium levels.

Dosage: One tablet, three times per day with meals.

Digestive Support

Zypan® (Standard Process): Provides betaine hydrochloride along with ammonium chloride to ensure gastric ionization of calcium.

Dosage: One to two tablets, three times per day with meals.

Parathyroid Support

Cal-Ma Plus® (Standard Process): This is desiccated parathyroid along with calcium and magnesium in the proper 5:1 ratio.

Dosage: One tablet, three times per day with meals for three months.

Kidney Support

Renafood® (Standard Process): Provides those nutrients and Protomorphogen™ extracts needed to ensure optimal kidney functioning.

Note: The kidneys convert 25 hydroxycholecalciferol (vitamin D) from the liver to its more active form. Without this occurring, the parathyroid hormone will not support calcium absorption from the intestinal tract.

Dosage: Two to three tablets, three times per day with meals. Can be used long term.

Liver Support: Refer to the section titled General Liver Support

Note: The liver is responsible for converting Vitamin D3 to 25 hydroxycholecalciferol. Without good liver function, vitamin D utilization will be compromised.

For low estrogen levels, consider one or more of the following as the case dictates.

1. **Wild Yam Complex (MediHerb):** Four to six tablets per day.
2. **Ovex® (Standard Process):** Two tablets three times per day.
3. **Tribulus (MediHerb):** One tablet three times per day.
4. **Black Cohosh 1:2 (MediHerb):** Three mL per day.
5. **White Peony 1:2 (MediHerb):** Seven mL per day.

Peptic Ulcers

Defined

Any disruption or irritation to the mucosal lining of the stomach, esophagus, or duodenum is termed a peptic ulcer. Of the three types, duodenal ulcers are the most common.

Symptoms

- Peptic ulcers can be asymptomatic
- Abdominal pain approximately 30-45 minutes after eating
- Abdominal pain at night
- Occult blood may be found in the stools in the case of bleeding ulcers

Etiology

Ulceration occurs when irritation from Helicobacter pylori, pepsin, or acid create damage to the mucosal lining.

The stomach and duodenum have a layer of mucopolysaccharides that coat their lining. This protects both areas from gastric secretions that have a pH of 1-3. The majority of people who have gastric ulcers have normal or reduced gastric secretions. Some people with duodenal ulcers exhibit an increase in gastric secretions. There are a small percentage of people who have an elevated number of parietal cells compared to the general population; however, the normal mucin coating should offer enough protection against this low pH secretion to compensate for the excess acid output. Excessive consumption of refined carbohydrates has been linked with increased hydrochloric acid production.

A loss of the mucilaginous protective layer could also be due to the following: Non Steroidal Anti-Inflammatory Drugs (NSAIDs), aspirin, alcohol overuse, toxins in the food, and inadequate intake of the nutritional factors needed to support synthesis of the mucopolysaccharides that line the gastric and duodenal regions.

Treatment Considerations

Consider the following when providing nutritional and/or herbal support with those who have peptic ulcers.

- Over colonization of Helicobacter Pylori has been found in 60-70% of those with a gastric ulcer and 90-95% of those with duodenal ulcers.
- NSAIDs can damage the gastric and duodenal mucosa.
- Aspirin has been linked to the formation gastric ulcers and not duodenal ulcers.
- Caffeine stimulates gastric acid production.
- There is an associated link between smoking and gastric ulcers.
- Insufficient pancreatic bicarbonate production can play a role in ulcer formation.
- Stress can play a role in ulcer formation.
- What is the integrity of the gastric mucosal lining? Is this lining healthy? Can it withstand the hydrochloric acid, pepsin, or other noxious compounds?
- Does the person in question have the ability to initiate and maintain a healing response to the damaged epithelial tissue?

Supplementation

When formulating a protocol, the following actions are desired:

- Anti-microbial
- Anti-inflammatory
- Immune support and/or stimulation

- Demulcent activity (soothing)
- Mucous membrane trophorestorative
- Vulnerary (wound healing)

Support needs to be continued until the practitioner feels that adequate healing has occurred. Patients with a peptic ulcer may need medical management in conjunction with natural therapies. **The potential for serious complications do exist with these conditions.**

Primary Support

Gastrex® (Standard Process): Supplies those factors needed to facilitate healing and cleansing of the upper gastrointestinal tract along with relief from the irritation of gastric acidity.

Dosage: Two capsules 15-20 minutes before meals.

HiPep Phytosynergist™ (MediHerb): The five herbs in this formula provide the following actions:

- Relieves the effects of gastric acidity
- Supports healing of the mucous membranes
- Provides demulcent and anti-inflammatory activity

Dosage: Five mL three times per day 15-20 minutes before meals.

Okra Pepsin E3 (Standard Process): Supplies those factors needed to facilitate healing and cleansing of the upper gastrointestinal tract.

Dosage: Two to three capsules three times per day between meals.

Dermatrophin PMG® (Standard Process): Support for the epithelial tissues as found in the digestive tract utilizing Protomorphogen™ extracts.

Dosage: One to two tablets three times per day with meals.

Secondary Support: As Indicated

Golden Seal 500mg (MediHerb): Anti-microbial support if Helicobacter pylori involvement is suspected. Mucous membrane trophorestorative and astringent.

Dosage: One tablet two times per day.

Licorice High Grade 1:1 (MediHerb): Encourages mucus secretion by the gastric mucosa and has anti-inflammatory and demulcent activity.

Dosage: Three mL per day.

Chlorophyll Complex™ (Standard Process): Counteracts gastric and intestinal inflammation, promotes healthy intestinal flora, and is a mucous membrane trophorestorative.

Dosage: Two to three perles three times per day. Best taken between meals.

Echinacea Premium (MediHerb): Immune system enhancement and anti-inflammatory.

Dosage: One tablet three times per day.

Aloe Vera 4.5:1 (MediHerb): Provides anti-inflammatory, immune enhancing, and vulnerary actions.

Dosage: Twenty-five mL two to three times per day before meals in addition to or in place of the primary support.

Polycystic Ovarian Syndrome (PCOS)

Defined

Polycystic Ovary Syndrome (PCOS) is an endocrine disorder in which the ovaries are slightly enlarged and contain multiple small cysts. This has led to the descriptive term, polycystic ovaries (also referred to as Stein-Leventhal syndrome, polycystic ovarian disease, or hyperandrogenic chronic anovulation). The definitive criteria for PCOS are cystic ovaries, secondary amenorrhea, and infertility as a result of anovulation. Lab findings will show mildly elevated androgens and a high LH (luteinizing hormone) to FSH (follicle stimulating hormone) ratio, lipid abnormalities (increased triglycerides), and insulin resistance.

Signs and Symptoms

A multifaceted hormonal disorder characterized by excessive production of androgens, increased levels of LH, and low levels of FSH. While the cause of PCOS is unknown, not all of these hormonal aberrations appear in all women. Some of the common presentations of patients with PCOS are:

- **Menstrual Irregularities:** A normal puberty and menarche, followed by episodes of amenorrhea that become progressively worse.
- **Infertility/SubFertility:** Irregular ovulation can make conceiving difficult. Similarly, if ovulation is not taking place (anovulation), it is not possible to conceive.
- **Hair and Skin Problems:** In PCOS the production of the androgen, testosterone, is excessive, causing abnormally increased hair growth (hirsutism) and contributes to acne formation.
- **Obesity:** About 50 percent of women with PCOS are obese.
- **Diabetes Mellitus:** Women with PCOS are more resistant to the action of insulin than normal women and, as a result, have a greater long-term risk of developing Metabolic Syndrome/Insulin Resistance.
- **Heart Disease:** Another long-term concern is that of cardiovascular risk. Androgens are known to induce an unfavorable lipid profile by increasing low density lipoprotein (LDL) and decreasing high density lipoprotein (HDL). Thus, the excessive production of androgen in PCOS may place these women at an increased risk for heart disease

Polycystic Ovarian Syndrome increases the risk of the following conditions:

- Miscarriage
- Heart disease
- Endometrial cancer

Etiology

The exact cause of PCOS is unknown. It was previously believed that PCOS was caused by excess androgen production. It has recently been shown that insulin resistance and hyperinsulinemia are core issues that, in turn; cause the overproduction of androgens by the ovaries. However, diverse causative factors could affect different women.

Treatment Considerations

- Address insulin resistance with diet and natural remedies
- Promote hormone balance
- Provide support for healthy uterine functioning
- Support normal ovulation
- Reduce luteinizing hormone
- Reduce androgen levels
- Support any emotional components (e.g. stress, anxiety)
- Institute a weight loss program if more than 10% over the desired BMI

Polycystic Ovarian Syndrome (PCOS)

Supplementation

Primary Support

White Peony 1:2 and Licorice 1:1 (MediHerb): The synergy of these two herbs act to support the ovaries and adrenal glands and help reduce high androgen production.

Dosage: White Peony – Four mL two times per day.
    And
    Licorice – Two mL two times per day.

Tribulus (MediHerb): The complex hormone balancing actions of this herb may help to restore normal ovarian function and fertility in women with PCOS.

Dosage: One tablet, three times per day on days 5 to 14 of the menstrual cycle.

Black Cohosh 1:2 (MediHerb): Estrogen modulating and a uterine tonic.

Dosage: Two mL per day upon rising to decrease LH levels.

Ovatrophin PMG® (Standard Process): Ovarian Protomorphogen™ extract support.

Dosage: One to two tablets three times per day with meals.

Secondary Support: As Indicated

Chaste Tree (MediHerb): Clinical evidence indicates this herb can assist in restoring hormone balance. In rare instances, Chaste Tree may aggravate PCOS, therefore careful monitoring of each case is advised.

Dosage: Two tablets upon rising.

COMMENT: Use of Chaste Tree is debated, but it may assist hormone balance.

Gymnema 4g or Gymnema 1:1 (both MediHerb): A bitter, antidiabetic, and hypoglycemic herb. Gymnema reduces the rate of absorption of simple sugars from the intestinal tract into the portal blood stream. The liquid has the additional benefit of helping to reduce the sense of taste for sweet foods.

Dosage: Gymnema 4g – One tablet, two times per day.
    Or
    Gymnema 1:1 – Four mL, three times per day.

Nevaton® (MediHerb): Nervine tonic addresses cases of PCOS that are aggravated by stress and depression.

Dosage: One tablet, three to four times per day.

LivCo® (MediHerb): To enhance hepatic clearance of endogenous estrogens and xenobiotics. Upregulates phase I cytochrome P450 and phase II liver detoxification mechanisms.

Dosage: One tablet, three times per day.

Clinical Notes

- Weight management patients can use the Standard Process Purification Program.
- Reduce sugar and hydrogenated fats, increase EFA's, complex carbohydrates, eating smaller, frequent meals to manage insulin resistance should also be addressed.

Premenstrual Syndrome

Defined

Premenstrual syndrome (PMS) refers to the recurring cyclical symptoms that occur during the luteal phase of the menstrual cycle.

Signs and Symptoms

Sufferers of PMS may experience any number of the following common symptoms.

- Spotting
- Heavy bleeding with or without cramping
- Clotting
- Acne
- Breast pain
- Infrequent or no menses
- Swelling/bloating
- Emotional (depression and/or anxiety)

- Decreased libido
- Mood swings
- Sugar cravings
- Headaches
- Gallbladder problems
- Hypoglycemia
- Muscle tension
- Cold hands and feet

Etiology

- In many clinical practices, estrogen dominance is a current theory that appears to deserve consideration. Estrogen dominance is not necessarily only the over-production of estrogen but also a decrease of the relative ratio of progesterone to estrogen during the luteal phase. During the luteal phase, progesterone should be the dominant hormone with respect to estrogen. A reduction in the ratio of progesterone to estrogen is defined as estrogen dominance.

Causes of Estrogen Dominance

- Hormone replacement therapy
- Nutritional deficiencies
- Xenoestrogen exposure

- Low-fiber diet
- Poor liver function
- Relative progesterone deficiency

Note: Estrogen dominance will be covered in this section along with the emotional issues associated with PMS. For other issues, such as adrenal fatigue and/or inadequate liver function, please refer to the appropriate individual topics in this manual.

- Over-production of prolactin has been indicated in PMS. Prolactin is produced by the anterior pituitary gland, and its levels can be influenced by stress. For example: a female under stress can secrete elevated levels of prolactin, producing a syndrome known as latent hyperprolactinemia. Latent hyperprolactinemia can be the cause of breast tenderness commonly experienced with PMS.

- An excess of adrenal hormones, cortisol, aldosterone, and epinephrine. One plausible explanation is a sub-optimal functioning liver that results in the body's inability to adequately breakdown and remove these endogenously produced hormones.

- Epinephrine, norepinephrine, dopamine, and serotonin also play a role in PMS. Epinephrine contributes to anxiety; norepinephrine is associated with irritability and hostility; dopamine promotes calmness and an increased ability to focus; whereas serotonin is associated with nervous tension. A high estrogen level is associated with increased levels of epinephrine, norepinephrine, and serotonin and lower levels of dopamine.

- Dopamine levels have an inverse relationship to prolactin levels. Low magnesium levels are also associated with lowered dopamine levels.

- An imbalance of pro-inflammatory prostaglandins to anti-inflammatory prostaglandins has also been implicated in PMS.

116

Premenstrual Syndrome

Treatment Considerations

Most women are not eating organic, and/or free-range foods. Couple this with xenobiotics that have estrogenic effects on the body, and the result is that most patients are going to be estrogen dominant. With this in mind, consideration must be given to balancing out the relative ratio of progesterone to estrogen during the luteal phase.

The following protocol can bring relief to PMS sufferers especially in cases of relative estrogen dominance. In practice, this protocol will address many of the PMS symptoms but not typically cramps. If cramps are an issue along with PMS, then Cramplex (see below) needs to be added to the protocol. If cramps are the only issue, then Chaste Tree is contraindicated. For this situation, use only Cramplex along with Ovatrophin PMG®.

Since emotions will affect the body physiologically as previous discussed, these symptoms need to also be addressed.

Supplementation

Primary Protocol

Black Currant Seed Oil (Standard Process): Rich source of gamma-linolenic acid (GLA). Many PMS patients are unable to convert linoleic acid to (GLA) – Black Currant Seed Oil, by providing pre-formed GLA, overcomes this deficit. The balance of essential fats found in Black Currant Seed Oil is of benefit in cases of PMS in order to mount an adequate anti-inflammatory response.

Dosage: Two perles, three times daily with meals.

Chaste Tree (MediHerb): Helps to increase LH levels and reduce excess prolactin levels. Overall effect is to ensure ovulation so that normal endogenous progesterone levels are maintained and to offset any relative estrogen dominance.

Dosage: One to two tablets per day preferably upon arising.

Clinical Notes: HRT and Chaste Tree

- *If the patient is on birth control agents or hormone replacement therapy in the form of estrogen and a synthetic progestin, then Chaste Tree is contraindicated. Use Ovex® at a dosage of one to two tablets three times per day with meals instead of Chaste tree.*
- *If patient is on estrogen alone, then use Chaste Tree.*
- *Chaste Tree, Ovex® and Ovaptrohpin PMG® can be used long term.*
- *If cramping is the only symptom, then do not use Chaste Tree because it will exacerbate the dysmennorhea. In this situation, use Cramplex instead as described below.*

Ovatrophin PMG® (Standard Process): Ovarian support utilizing *Protomorphogen*™ extracts.

Dosage: One to two tablets three times per day with meals.

Note: *Use the list below to recommend a remedy once you have determined which of the following emotional components may need nutritional and/or herbal support. Remember, in practice if you do not address the emotional factors, it may be more difficult to obtain the desired positive clinical outcome.*

PMS with depression and anxiety:

Nevaton (MediHerb): The combination of herbs in this formula are effective for the symptoms of depression and anxiety. It also supports liver detoxification of both endogenously produced estrogen and exogenous xenoestrogens.

Dosage: One tablet, three to four times per day.

Premenstrual Syndrome

PMS with depression alone:

St. John's Wort 1.8g (MediHerb): For mild to moderate depression. Up regulates both phase I and II of the cytochrome P450 mixed function oxidase system in the liver. This results in increased detoxification and subsequent excretion of endogenously produced estrogens and exogenous xenoestrogens.

Dosage: One tablet, three to four times per day.

PMS with fatigue:

Withania Complex (MediHerb): Wonderful formula for those who are hyped-up and fatigued at the same time. Indicated where adrenal fatigue is suspected.

Dosage: One tablet, three to four times per day.

And/or

Valerian Complex (MediHerb): For those who suffer from a combination of fatigue and nervous tension.

Dosage: One tablet, three to four times per day.

Note: Regarding the primary protocol, allow at least three cycles to see the maximum benefit of the remedies prescribed.

Secondary Protocol: If Indicated

PMS with edema:

Dandelion Leaves 1:1 (MediHerb): Diuretic action to help with weight gain, swollen ankles and/or swollen abdomen associated with excess fluid retention. Dandelion leaf is very high in potassium and will not deplete the body of potassium as is the case with many diuretics.

Dosage: Five mL twice a day.

PMS with pain:

E.g., lower back pain, reduced pain threshold (due to prostaglandins)

Boswellia Complex (MediHerb): The synergistic effects of the herbs in this formula reduce inflammation and facilitate the removal of metabolic acids.

Dose: One to two tablets, three times per day.

Saligesic (MediHerb): Provides analgesic and anti-inflammatory activity.

Dose: Mild Pain: One tablet twice daily.
Severe Pain: One tablet four times daily.

PMS with menstrual cramping:

Cramplex (MediHerb): Relieves pain, inflammation, and uterine spasm associated with period pain.

Dosage: Two tablets, every three to four hours up to eight per day as noted below.

Cramplex can be used on an as needed basis during the menstrual cycle. A day or two before menses have the patient take two tablets every three to four hours up to eight per day. Once the cramps subside, discontinue the Cramplex and resume monthly as prescribed.

Prenatal Nutrition

Defined

Prenatal nutrition includes providing nutrients to support development of a healthy baby and the well-being of the mother.

Prenatal supplementation is necessary today due to the effects of the typical diet of overly processed, chemically adulterated, genetically modified, and irradiated food. Supplementation is needed during pregnancy to make up for deficiencies this type of diet creates.

Good prenatal nutrition is critical for the health of future generations. Weston Price, D.D.S. noted while studying different cultures, that it takes only one generation of eating poorly (Western diet) to compromise the health of the offspring. Synthetic prenatal vitamins cannot fill the gap created by a poor diet.

Supplementation

Primary Support

Catalyn® (Standard Process): Multiple vitamin and major mineral source along with naturally occurring food enzymes. Formulated from whole food sources, processed with low heat and only the fiber and moisture removed, Catalyn® supplies multiple essential food factors to provide general nutritional foundational support.

Dosage: Two to three tablets, three times per day with meals.

Note: For the benefits of Catalyn® together with naturally occurring fiber, consider using Cyrofood® from Standard Process (4 tablets three times per day with meals) or Cyrofood® Powder (one to two tablespoons three times per day mixed with water and fruit in a blender).

Folic Acid B12 (Standard Process): A synergistic formula to support neural tube formation in the early developing fetus (prior to 6 weeks) and CNS development thereafter.

Dosage: One to two tablets, three times per day with meals.

Calcium Lactate (Standard Process): A growing baby needs considerable amount of calcium during development. If the baby is not getting enough to meet its needs, the body will release calcium from the bones (most of the calcium in the body is inside bones) to meet the baby's requirements. Inadequate dietary calcium intake during pregnancy can increase the risk for osteoporosis later in life for the mother. Calcium lactate provides a readily available form of calcium balanced with magnesium to supplement a diet high in green leafy vegetables during this time of increased requirements.

Dosage: Four tablets, three times per day on an empty stomach for maximum absorption.

Some Non-Dairy Sources of Calcium

- Almonds
- Broccoli
- Beet greens
- Kale
- Mustard greens
- Bok Choy
- Spinach
- Mackerel
- Kelp
- Canned salmon with soft bones

Prenatal Nutrition

For women who will not eat sufficient quantities of vegetables, consider one or more of the following:

1. **Cruciferous Complete™ (Standard Process):** Combination of Kale and Brussels sprouts. Kale is a rich source of the vitamin C complex, beta-carotene, chlorophyll, vitamin E complex, and trace minerals along with the known and unknown phytochemicals. Brussels sprouts are also a rich source of vitamin C, iron, vitamin A, folic acid, potassium, and phytochemicals.

   Dosage: One to two capsules, three times daily with meals.

2. **Betafood® (Standard Process):** Each tablet is composed of beet root and leaf. The root is source of folic acid, potassium, betaine (excellent liver support) and the greens are a rich source of beta-carotene, calcium, and iron. Both the root and leaf supply vitamin C along with those critical phytonutrients and antioxidants needed to ensure optimum health.

   Dosage: Two tablets, three times daily with meals.

3. **SP Green Food™ (Standard Process):** Brussels sprouts, kale, alfalfa, buckwheat juice powder (high source of magnesium, the bioflavonoid rutin, and a source of essential amino acids), barley grass juice powder (supplies niacin, iron, magnesium, manganese, phosphorous, selenium, and zinc), and alfalfa sprout powder (trace mineral and vitamin K source).

   Dosage: One capsule, three times daily with meals.

Ferrofood® (Standard Process): Provides those factors, including ferrous lactate, needed to support healthy red blood cell production. This is a blood building formula which includes iron.

Dosage: One capsule, three times per day with meals.

Linum B6 (Standard Process): Source of Omega 3 and Omega 6 essential fatty acids.

Dosage: Two perles, two to three times per day with meals.

Secondary Support: As Indicated

If a pregnant woman will not take a lot of supplements, recommend the following two products.

Immuplex® (Standard Process): Given in conjunction with Catalyn® (6-9 tablets per day) to ensure that the mother does not become depleted during pregnancy. Provides the vitamin A, C, and E complexes, folic acid, cyanocobalamin, trace minerals, and liver, thymus, spleen, and bone Protomorphogen™ extracts along with other synergistic factors for optimal immune system support.

Dosage: Two to three capsules three times per day with meals.

Cataplex® G (Standard Process): Supplies additional B-complex vitamins including vitamin B12, Glucose Tolerance Factor, amino acids, and trace minerals.

Dosage: Two to three tablets, three times per day with meals.

Sinusitis (Acute, Chronic)

Defined

Sinusitis is an inflammatory process in the paranasal sinuses. Etiological factors can be bacterial, viral, fungal infections, or allergic reactions. Sinusitis may occur in any of the four groups of sinuses: ethmoid, frontal, sphenoid, or maxillary.

Signs and Symptoms

- Pain and tenderness over the effected sinus
- Headaches
- Nasal congestion
- Postnasal drip

- Malaise
- Nasal discharge of yellow or green pus
- Fever and chills
- Reduced sense of smell

Etiology

A viral upper respiratory tract infection usually precedes the onset of an acute bacterial sinusitis. Other etiological causes can include an underlying dental infection, food allergies, pollution, tobacco smoke, dust, powder or chemical exposure from the work environment, allergic rhinitis, and a compromised immune system. Any of these factors can cause a swelling of the sinus mucous membranes with resultant stasis of drainage and subsequent bacterial infection.

Acute sinusitis episodes can be recurrent; however, sinusitis can be considered chronic if the symptoms persist for more than three months.

Treatment Considerations

- Reduced sense of smellImmune support with nutritional supplementation and/or herbs
- Anticatarrhal agents to reduce stasis
- Mucolytic herbs to reduce stasis
- Removal of environmental agents and foods that stimulate excessive mucus production

pplementation

Primary Support: Acute Sinusitis

plex® A-C (Standard Process): Source of the vitamin A and C complexes, both of which are necessary to nize connective tissue healing and support immune functioning.

age: Four tablets, three times per day with meals during the acute phase. Reduce the dosage to two tablets three times per day for long term healing.

: Consider the addition of **Cal-Amo®** (Standard Process) at a dosage of two tablets, three times per day to acidify the involved alkaline tissues.

rasia Complex (MediHerb): The overall effects of the herbs in this formula are to reduce mucus secretions the nasal passages and to strengthen and tone the mucous membranes.

Dosage: Two tablets, three times per day.

Sinusitis (Acute, Chronic)

Golden Seal 500mg (MediHerb): A trophorestorative herb for the mucous membranes with anticatarrhal, antimicrobial, antibacterial, and anti-inflammatory properties.

Dosage: One tablet, two to three times per day. Very good when the secretions are green and/or yellow.

Primary Support: Chronic Sinusitis

Euphrasia Complex (MediHerb): The overall effects of the herbs in this formula reduce the allergic response, reduce mucus secretion of the nasal passages, and strengthen and tone the mucous membranes.

Dosage: One tablet, three to four times per day.

Andrographis Complex (MediHerb): Especially useful for acute conditions of the upper respiratory tract. A good formula used to boost immunity for any bacterial infection or disorder characterized by low immunity.

Dosage: One tablet, three to four times per day. For very acute conditions, consider two tablets three to four times per day.

Secondary Support for Acute and Chronic Sinusitis: As Indicated

Albizia Complex (MediHerb): An anti-allergic formula that can be used with Euphrasia Complex where allergies are the main cause of sinusitis. The overall effect of this formula is to reduce inflammation, provide relief of allergic symptoms, and provide anti-microbial support.

Dosage: One tablet, three to four times per day.

Fen-Gre® (Standard Process): Each capsule supplies 270 mg fenugreek seed powder, a mucolytic herb. Add to primary support if mucus discharge is thick and does not drain easily from the sinuses.

Dosage: Three capsules, three times per day with a full glass of water if used without Euphrasia complex. One capsule, three times per day with a full glass of water when used with Euphrasia complex.

Sprains and Strains

Defined and Etiology

A sprain is an injury to a joint in which some of the fibers of a supporting ligament are ruptured but the continuity of the ligament remains intact.

A strain is the overstretching or overexertion of some part of the musculature.

Symptoms

- Pain
- Swelling
- Reduced mobility
- Muscular spasms

Treatment Considerations

- Provide nutritional support to support soft tissue and ligamentous healing
- Use of anti-edema agents and anti-inflammatory herbs

Supplementation

The following products should all be considered when dealing with a sprain/strain type injury. It is recommended that one use Ligaplex® II as a foundation, and recommend the other products as the case warrants.

Ligaplex® I (Standard Process): Source of vitamin A, C, and E complexes, B12, phosphorous, manganese, connective tissue Protomorphogen™ extract, ribonucleic acid, and liver powder. This combination of nutrients, as other nutrients contained within this formula synergistically provides the factors to support ligament and soft tissue healing.

Dosage: Three capsules, three times per day with meals.

Cataplex® A-C (Standard Process): Source of the vitamin A and C complex factors, both of which have a role in tissue regeneration and collagen formation.

Dosage: Two to three tablets, three times per day with meals.

Boswellia Complex (MediHerb): Anti-inflammatory herbal blend which reduces leukotriene formation and supports removal of metabolic acids.

Dosage: Four to six tablets per day depending on severity of symptoms.

Horsechestnut Complex (MediHerb): Herbal formula containing Horsechestnut, Butcher's Broom, and *Gingko* which help to reduce edema and congestion.

Dosage: One tablet, two to three times per day.

Note: Patients should continue on the nutritional and/or herbal remedies until the practitioner feels adequate results have taken place.

Tinnitus (Ringing in Ears)

Defined

Tinnitus is defined as a noise in the ears, which can manifest as a ringing, buzzing, roaring, or clicking sound.

Symptoms

- Chronic noise in the ears

Etiology

Some researchers make a distinction between vibratory and non-vibratory tinnitus. This may have value etiologically.

- Non-vibratory tinnitus is considered a biochemical change in the auditory nerve
- Vibratory tinnitus may indicate a mechanical problem with hearing

Other factors that can affect hearing are:

- Ear drum disruption induced tinnitus
- Middle ear infections
- Eustacian tube blockage induced tinnitus (sinus and allergy problems included)
- Noise induced tinnitus (cochlea damage)
- Auditory nerve damage induced tinnitus
- High cholesterol induced tinnitus
- Stress, shock or trauma induced tinnitus
- Viral infections (Herpes zoster oticus) induced tinnitus
- TMJ (Temporo-Mandibular Joint) induced tinnitus
- Hyperacusis – reduced tolerance to sounds (normal, everyday noises are too loud)
- Meniere's Disease – symptoms are vertigo, nausea, dizziness and tinnitus
- Thyroid disease
- Drug induced auditory nerve damage (aspirin, anti-inflammatory drugs, antibiotics, and antidepressants)
- Otosclerosis (stiffening of the joints formed by the small bones of the ear, i.e. stapes, incus and malleus)
- High blood pressure or circulatory problems inducing tinnitus

Treatment Considerations

- Improve blood flow and oxygenation to auditory apparatus
- Enhance immunity
- Reduce cholesterol

Special Note: This is one of those conditions where a positive clinical outcome may be difficult to achie for causes other than infection and cholesterol buildup in the tubes of the ear.

Tinnitus (Ringing in Ears)

Supplementation

Primary Support: Cholesterol Buildup

Cyruta® (Standard Process): Combination of inositol (lipotrophic factor) and buckwheat leaf and seed juice (choline source) along with synergistic factors that encourage blood flow and blood fat transport. Buckwheat is a rich source of rutin, a bioflavonoid that has a critical role in maintaining capillary wall integrity.

Dosage: Two to three tablets, three times per day with meals.

Cataplex® G (Standard Process): Source of B vitamin complex to support vasodilation. Lipotrophic factors are also contained in Cataplex® G to facilitate the liver's handling of fats, including cholesterol

Dosage: Two tablets, three times per day with meals.

Ginkgo 2000mg (MediHerb): Circulatory stimulant.

Dosage: Two tablets, twice per day.

Primary Support: Middle Ear Infections

See the section titled *Middle Ear Infection* for additional information and protocols.

Varicose Veins

Defined

Elongated, tortuous, dilated superficial veins (usually in the legs) with incompetent valves that permit reversed flow.

Symptoms

- Initially, superficial veins that are varicosed may be tense and palpable but not necessarily visible. They may later enlarge and protrude and then become visibly obvious.
- Small varicosities may be painful whereas severe leg involvement may be asymptomatic.
- Aching, fatigue, or heat in the legs which is relieved by leg elevation.

- Heavy feeling in the legs.
- Restless legs in bed.
- Edema in ankles.
- Discoloration with or without ulceration.
- Itch in lower leg and ankle.

Etiology

- Nutritional deficiency resulting in a weakness of the vein walls
- Obesity
- Prolonged standing aggravates varicose veins and can be an etiologic factor if the veins are weak to begin with
- Hormonal changes during pregnancy and increased pressure on the pelvic veins later in pregnancy
- Abdominal tumor
- Hepatic portal hypertension
- Congenital arteriovenous fistulas

Treatment Considerations

Natural remedies can be of help in improving vein function and relieving the symptoms of varicose veins. Larg[e] varicosities may not remit; however, it is possible to prevent continued venous deterioration. The following a[ctions] are desired when providing nutritional and herbal support for varicose veins:

- Vasoprotection
- Antioxidant
- Anti-inflammatory
- Astringent

- Venotonic
- Collagen stabilizing
- Circulatory stimulant

Supplementation

Primary Support

Horsechestnut Complex (MediHerb): Combination of Horsechestnut, Feverfew, and Butcher's Broom provides anti-inflammatory, venotonic, antioxidant, circulatory stimulant, collagen stabilizing, and vasoprotection.

Dosage: One tablet, two to three times per day.

Biost® (Standard Process): Connective tissue Protomorphogen™ extract support.

Dosage: Two tablets, three times per day with meals.

OPC Synergy™ (Standard Process): Containing Masquelier's Original OPC antioxidant formula, OPC Synergy combines grape seed extract, buckwheat, red wine extract, green tea extract, and bilberry to provide oligoproanthocyanadins, which improve microcirculation and provide additional antioxidant, venotonic, astringent, and anti-inflammatory support.

Dosage: One tablet, two to three times per day with meals.

Bilberry 6000mg (MediHerb): Provides additional vasoprotective, antioxidant, anti-inflammatory, and astringent actions.

Dosage: One tablet, three to four times per day.

Secondary Support: As Indicated

Collinsonia Root (Standard Process): Also called Stone Root has been used traditionally as a vascular astringent, thus it helps maintain proper tone in the vascular system.

Dosage: Two to three capsules twice daily with a full glass of water between meals.

Cyruta® Plus (Standard Process): Rich source of rutin, which provides those factors needed to stabilize weak blood vessels and reduce capillary fragility.

Dosage: One to three tablets, three times per day with a full glass of water.

Viral Hepatitis (Acute)

Defined

A group of several forms of hepatitis caused by viruses resulting in inflammation of the liver.

Signs and Symptoms

The liver is the second largest organ (after the skin) of the body and participates in functions associated with the cardiovascular system, digestive system, excretory system and metabolism. Therefore, any condition that compromises liver function can result in varied and diverse symptomatology. With this in mind, acute viral hepatitis can produce anything from minor flu-like symptoms to fatal liver failure. Clinicians should be aware of the many symptoms that are possible besides the ones listed below.

The following are some of the more **common** symptoms that occur with hepatitis.

- Fatigue
- Joint pain
- Loss of appetite
- Dark urine
- Diarrhea
- Fever
- Jaundice
- Tender enlarged liver
- Light colored stools
- Itching
- Headache

- Muscle pain
- Abdominal pain
- Nausea
- Vomiting

Etiology

Hepatitis (inflammation of the liver) is usually (but not always) caused by viruses. The most common viral causes include hepatitis A (non-enveloped virus), hepatitis B (enveloped virus), and hepatitis C (enveloped virus). Other forms of viral hepatitis are those caused by Cytomegalovirus, Epstein-Barr, Herpes simplex, and hepatitis virus D (enveloped) and E (non-enveloped).

The hepatitis viruses are transmitted as follows:

- **Hepatitis A:** Spread via fecal contamination in the food or water. Can also be spread via blood.
- **Hepatitis B:** Spread via blood, blood products, and sexual contact. This virus is found in semen, saliv vaginal secretions. Another possible route of transmission is by way of mother to child.
- **Hepatitis C:** Similar transmission to Hepatitis B.
- **Hepatitis D:** This virus can only infect a carrier of Hepatitis B.
- **Hepatitis E:** Transmitted via oral-fecal route.

Hepatitis A, B, C, D, and E usually will not develop into a chronic condition. Hepatitis A usually remits in tv three months and Hepatitis B, C, D, and E in four to five months.

Chronic hepatitis occurs in 5 to 10 percent of those with Hepatitis B and can occur in up to 50 percent of those with Hepatitis C. Chronic viral hepatitis can be asymptomatic or lead to severe liver damage, liver cancer, and even death.

Viral Hepatitis (Acute)

Treatment Considerations

Whole food concentrates and herbs that are recommended provide the following actions as indicated:

- Immune enhancement and modulation
- Hepatoprotection
- Hepatotrophorestorative
- Antiviral for the specific type of virus
- Diaphoretic

Supplementation

Primary Support

Andrographis Complex (MediHerb): This formula is immune enhancing and hepatoprotective through the combined effects of Andrographis, Echinacea, and Holy Basil.

Dosage: Two tablets, two to three times a day.

Hepatrophin PMG® (Standard Process): Liver support utilizing Protomorphogen™ extracts.

Dosage: One to two tablets, three times per day with meals.

Silymarin (MediHerb): The flavonolignans in Milk Thistle provide hepatoprotective, hepatotrophorestorative, and choleretic activity.

Dosage: Two tablets, two times per day.

St John's Wort 1.8g (MediHerb): Acts as an antiviral agent specifically against enveloped viruses.

Dosage: Two tablets, two times per day.

Note: This protocol and corresponding doses are to be used during the acute phase. Once the acute phase is over, long-term liver support is strongly recommended. Refer to the section titled *General Liver Support* for further dosage information.

Secondary Support: As Indicated

fever

Phytosynergist™ (MediHerb): The herbs in this formula provide anti-infective and immune enhancing along with fever modulation.

Four mL four times a day with warm water during the febrile phase.

al Antioxidant Protection for the Liver

gy™ (Standard Process): Rich source of antioxidants such as green tea extract, red wine extract, extract, bilberry, buckwheat, and carrot powder to provide additional hepatocyte protection.

One capsule, two to three times per day with meals.

dditional Liver Support: As Indicated

Livaplex® (Standard Process): The combined action of A-F Betafood®, Betacol®, Antronex®, Spanish Black Radish, Chezyn®, and Hepatrophin PMG® provides the factors that are needed to support healthy bile production and flow, bowel detoxification, liver decongestion through the use of to lipotrophic factors, hepatic Protomorphogen™ extract support, and enhanced blood flow through the portal vein.

Dosage: Two to three capsules, three times per day with meals.

Viral Hepatitis (Acute)

The following products provide the nutrients that are needed to support both optimal hepatocyte function and hepatic cellular detoxification processes.

Cruciferous Complete™ (Standard Process): Made from Kale and Brussels sprouts, both of which are a rich source of phytonutrients supportive of phase II liver detoxification pathways.

Dosage: One capsule, two to three times per day with meals.

Betafood® (Standard Process): Beet root and leaf. The betaine in red beets is a source of methyl donors which is supportive of phase II liver detoxification pathways. Beet leaf and root provide the nutritional factors to support healthy bile production and flow.

Dosage: One to two tablets, three times per day with meals.

Folic Acid B12 (Standard Process): Supports methylation of phase II liver detoxification.

Dosage: One tablet, two to three times per day with meals.

Garlic *(Organically Grown)* (Standard Process): The sulfur in garlic supports sulphation of the phase II liver detoxification pathway.

Dosage: One tablet, two to three times per day with meals.

Spanish Black Radish (Standard Process): Each tablet supplies 360 mg of Spanish Black Radish. Spanish black radish is a rich source of sulfur containing compounds which will be supportive of phase II liver detoxification pathways.

Dosage: Two tablets, three times per day with meals.

All the products listed in the secondary protocol can be used long term. With the typical American diet, most people are simply not eating the foods that support optimal liver functioning, much less getting enough nutrients to meet their bodies' demand. With this in mind, it would be wise to have your patient complete a seven-day food diary. This enables you to see what they aren't eating as well as what they are eating. If they are not eating, or will not eat kale, red beets, etc., then a recommendation to use one or more of the above long term should be considered.

Viral Hepatitis (Chronic)

Defined

An inflammation of the liver caused by a viral infection, usually Hepatitis B or C.

There are two main forms of chronic viral hepatitis:

1. Chronic persistent hepatitis – a benign condition
2. Chronic active hepatitis – a serious disorder that can result in liver failure and/or cirrhosis

Etiology/Symptoms

Chronic Persistent Hepatitis

- Typically follows acute hepatitis.
- Persistent high aminotransferase values with no or vague symptoms are characteristic. Jaundice is uncommon and liver function tests are usually unremarkable. Diagnosis is usually dependent on needle biopsy.

Chronic Active Hepatitis

- Usually the sequalae of infection with hepatitis B or C.
- Most cases of chronic active hepatitis are of unknown etiology with many of these cases having prominent autoimmune features.
- Can result in liver failure and/or cirrhosis.

Treatment Considerations

The goal of managing chronic viral hepatitis is to protect the liver from further damage, restore the integrity of the damaged hepatic tissue, and control the viral load.

- Long term immune system support is important in the management of chronic viral hepatitis. In this way, treatment will mirror that of acute viral hepatitis.
- Extended use of hepatic Protomorphogen™ extracts.
- Dietary counseling on nutritional habits to support the liver.
- Use of hepatoprotective and hepatotrophorestorative agents.
- Use of antiviral agents.
- Use of antioxidants to provide additional hepatocyte protection.

Supplementation

Primary Support

All of the following products can be used long term.

Hepatrophin PMG® (Standard Process): Liver support utilizing liver Protomorphogen™ extracts.

Dosage: One tablet, three times per day with meals.

Silymarin (MediHerb): The flavonolignans in Milk Thistle provide hepatoprotective, hepatotrophorestorative, and choleretic activity.

Dosage: One tablet, three to four times per day.

Echinacea Premium (MediHerb): Provides immune enhancing, anti-inflammatory, and depurative actions.

Dosage: One tablet, three times per day.

St John's Wort 1.8g (MediHerb): Antiviral agent, specifically active against enveloped viruses.

Dosage: One tablet, three to four times per day.

Livaplex® (Standard Process): Source of lipotrophic factors along with those nutrients needed to support bile production and flow as well as hepatic detoxification pathways.

Dosage: Two to three capsules, three times per day with meals.

Note: *It is imperative that patients with hepatitis eat foods that support hepatic function so the liver can carry out the myriad of tasks for which it is responsible. The following list of foods is important for nutrient support of the liver and should be eaten on a regular basis and prepared correctly.*

- *Fresh red beets- both the root and greens*
- *Broccoli*
- *Kale*
- *Cabbage*
- *Brussels sprouts*
- *Garlic*
- *Red peppers*
- *Onions*
- *Asparagus*

Secondary Support: As Indicated

For those who do not eat correctly, consider recommending any combination of the following depending on the individual case.

Betafood® (Standard Process): Beet root and leaf. The betaine in red beets is a source of methyl donors which is supportive of phase II liver detoxification pathways. Beet leaf and root provide the nutritional factors to support healthy bile production and flow.

Dosage: One to two tablets, three times per day with meals.

Cruciferous Complete™ (Standard Process): Made from Kale and Brussels sprouts, both of which are a rich source of phytonutrients supportive of phase II liver detoxification pathways.

Dosage: One capsule, two to three times per day with meals.

Spanish Black Radish (Standard Process): Each tablet supplies 360 mg of Spanish Black Radish. Spanish black radish is a rich source of sulfur containing compounds which will be supportive of phase II liver detoxification pathways.

Dosage: Two tablets, three times per day with meals.

Garlic (Organically Grown) (Standard Process): The sulfur in garlic supports sulphation of the phase II detoxification.

Dosage: One tablet, two to three times per day with meals.

Folic Acid B12 (Standard Process): Supports methylation of phase II liver detoxification.

Dosage: One tablet, two to three times per day.

OPC Synergy™ (Standard Process) or Vitanox (MediHerb): Antioxidant support to help protect and maintain integrity of the hepatocytes.

Dosage: One capsule, two to three times a day with meals.

Bibliography

Atlas of Pathophysiology. Springhouse Corporation and Anatomical Chart Company, 2002.

Beers, M., and R. Berkow. *The Merck Manual of Diagnostic & Therapy.* 17th ed. Whitehouse Station: Merck Research Labs, 1999.

Berkow, R., and M.B. Fletcher. T*he Merck Manual.* 16th ed. Rahway: Merck Research Lab, 1992.

Bone, Kerry. *Clinical Applications of Ayervedic and Chinese Herbs: Monographs written for the Western Herbal Practitioner.* Queensland, Australia: Phytotherapy Press, 1996.

Champe, P.C., and R. Harvey. *Biochemistry.* 2nd ed. Philadelphia: Lippincott, Williams & Wilkens, 1994.

Cotran, R., V. Kumar, and T. Collins. *Pathologic Basis of Disease.* 6th ed. Philadelphia: WB Saunders Co., 1999.

Crook, W.C. *The Yeast Connection.* New York: Vintage Books, 1986.

DeGowin, R., and D. Brown. *DeGowin's Diagnostic Examination.* 7th ed. New York: McGraw-Hill, 2000.

Duke, J. *The Green Pharmacy Herbal Handbook.* Rodale Inc, 2000.

Duke, J.A. *Phytochemical Constituents of GRAS Herbs and Other Economic Plants.* Boca Raton: CRC Press, 2001.

iedman, P.J. *Biochemistry.* 4th ed. Boston: Little, Brown & Co, 1992.

an, R. *Optimal Wellness.* New York: Ballantine Books, 1995.

ton, A.C. *Textbook of Medical Physiology.* 6th ed. Philadelphia: WB Saunders Co., 1981.

el, R. *Physiology Secrets.* Philadelphia: Hanley & Belfus Inc., 1999.

ann, G., and J. Kirschmann. *Nutrition Almanac.* 4th ed. New York City: McGraw-Hill, 1996.

, W. *Complementary & Alternative Medicine Secrets.* Philadelphia: Hanley & Belfus, 2002.

R. Cotran, and S. Robbins. *Basic Pathology*. 6th ed. Philadelphia: WB Saunders Co., 1997.

A.D. Marks, and C.M. Smith. *Basic Medical Biochemistry.* Philadelphia: Lippincott Williams & Wilkins, 1996.

and Kerry Bone. *Principles and Practice of Phytotherapy Modern Herbal Medicine.* Edinburgh: Churchill one, 2000.

ay, M., and J. Pizzorno. *Encyclopedia of Natural Medicine.* Rev. 2nd ed. Roseville: Prima Publishing, 1998.

rray, Michael, N.D., and Beutler Jade. *Understanding Fats and Oils: A Guide to Healing with Essential Fatty Acids.* Vancouver: Apple Publishing, 1996.

Nick, Gina, Ph.D, N.D. *Clinical Purification.* Brookfield: Longevity Through Prevention, 2001.

Pizzorno, J., and M. Murray. *Textbook of Natural Medicine.* 2nd ed. Vol I & II. London: Churchill Livingstone, 2000.

Bibliography

Pritchford, P. *Healing with Whole Foods.* Berkeley: North Atlantic Books, 1993.

Saunders. *Dorland's Illustrated Medical Dictionary*. 28th ed. Philadelphia: WB Saunders Co., 1994.

Sherman, H.C., and S.L. Smith. *The Vitamins.* 2nd ed. New York City: The Chemical Catalog Co. Inc., 1931.

Tips, J. *Candida and Restore Your Immune System.* Austin: Apple-A-Day Press, 2000.

Notes

Notes